POPULATION SCIENCE METHODS AND APPROACHES TO AGING AND ALZHEIMER'S DISEASE AND RELATED DEMENTIAS RESEARCH

POPULATION SCIENCE METHODS AND APPROACHES TO AGING AND ALZHEIMER'S DISEASE AND RELATED DEMENTIAS RESEARCH

EDITED BY

CHAU TRINH-SHEVRIN

JB JOSSEY-BASS™

A Wiley Brand

Library of Congress Cataloging-in-Publication Data
Names: Trinh-Shevrin, Chau- editor.
Title: Population science methods and approaches to aging and Alzheimer's disease and related dementias research / edited by Chau Trinh-Shevrin.
Description: Hoboken, NJ : John Wiley & Sons Inc., [2024] | Includes bibliographical references and index.
Identifiers: LCCN 2023026146 (print) | LCCN 2023026147 (ebook) | ISBN 9781394204144 (paperback) | ISBN 9781394204168 (adobe pdf) | ISBN 9781394204151 (epub)
Subjects: LCSH: Aging--Psychological aspects. | Alzheimer's disease. | Dementia.
Classification: LCC BF724.55.A35 P67 2023 (print) | LCC BF724.55.A35 (ebook) | DDC 155.67--dc23/eng/20230927
LC record available at https://lccn.loc.gov/2023026146
LC ebook record available at https://lccn.loc.gov/2023026147

Cover image: © Irina_QQQ/Shutterstock
Cover design: Thalassa Tam

Set in 10/12pt Times LT Std by Integra Software Services Pvt. Ltd, Pondicherry, India

SKY10064831_011324

CONTENTS

FIGURES AND TABLES

FIGURES

TABLES

PREFACE

> *The energy of the mind is the essence of life.*
> *–Aristotle*
>
> *The way you think, the way you behave, the way you eat, can influence your life by 30 to 50 years.*
> *–Deepak Chopra*

Aging begins at birth. Yet most people only begin to recognize and struggle with the aging process when they observe and experience a loss of their own youthful vitality, the breakdown of their bodies, and changes in their appearances. The effects of aging become more apparent to us as we watch our parents and loved ones endure advancing chronic conditions, comorbidities, isolation, and heightened vulnerability. In parallel, we see the reflection of these effects within our neighborhoods, communities, and society at large, producing new challenges for families and caregivers, health care providers, researchers, and policymakers. While national policies and programs, such as Medicare, are pivoting to become more cognizant and inclusive of aging-related conditions and the treatments and support needed by aging Americans and their care partners, there is an urgent need to focus attention and investment on population health approaches to address the unmet needs, sociocultural contexts, and health trajectories of older people.

While a vast array of aging-related conditions can impact the daily activities and well-being of older people, Alzheimer's disease and Alzheimer's disease-related dementias (AD/ADRD) are among the most feared of these conditions. These diagnoses portend a complete loss of self, including one's own identity, purpose, and autonomy as well as one's loss of self in relation to others. Profound memory loss eats away the connectedness of relationships spanning decades, rendering loved ones strangers – and, at times, strangers to be feared. As AD/ADRD advances, acute fear gives way to chronic anxiety, anger, and withdrawal. Caregivers of people living with AD/ADRD may find the most painful aspects of this process to be observing their loved ones suffer and become mere shells of the people they once were. It is important to distinguish dementia from AD. Dementia is not a specific disease; rather, it is a term that describes a set of symptoms including memory loss and confusion as well as the breakdown of daily life functioning and the ability to communicate and interact with others. AD is the most common cause of dementia, accounting for about 70% of patients diagnosed with dementia. Other forms of dementia include vascular dementia, dementia with Lewy bodies, frontotemporal dementia, Cruetzfeldt-Jakob disease, Huntington's disease, normal pressure hydrocephalus, and mixed dementia (i.e., a combination of two or more sources of dementia). Typically, this group of diseases is referred to as AD/ADRD. In addition to degenerative diseases, like AD or Parkinson's disease, other causes of dementia may include chronic drug use, depression, infections, stroke, and vascular disease. For some causes of dementia, there may be treatments to reverse cognitive impairment or slow down the progression of dementia symptoms. AD is a disease of the brain and is progressively degenerative, impairing areas of the brain that include learning, thinking, and bodily functioning and leading to debilitation over time. AD is currently irreversible.

Over the last two decades, there have been increasing and substantial investments in identifying and testing therapeutics to treat and potentially reverse AD. For example, researchers have focused on the role of plaque-forming beta-amyloid in the brain in accelerating AD-associated deterioration, leading to the development of monoclonal antibodies to the immune system to help clear beta-amyloid from the brain. An example of this type of drug is lecanamab (i.e., Lequembi), which received accelerated approval by the United States (US) Federal Drug Administration (FDA) in early 2023; previously, aducanemab (i.e., Aduhelm) was approved in 2021. Evidence from available trials does not yet establish definitively the effectiveness of these drugs in improving cognition (Ackley et al., 2021). Other drugs in development focus on preventing destruction of synapses and halting memory loss (e.g., saracatinib), while still others focus on blocking production of beta-amyloid (i.e., beta- and gamma-secretase inhibitors). None of these currently available therapies, however, has proven beneficial to all of the individuals who have participated in drug trials or to those who have been given these therapies in health care settings, indicating the need for more investment and focused research to better understand the mechanisms and expression of AD.

Increasingly, researchers and advocates are raising attention to the role of prevention and social factors in healthy aging. For example, the role of the microbiome and the significance of the mind–gut relationship have been demonstrated to influence the risk for depression, anxiety, and dementia. What we eat and the health of the microbial environment in our digestive systems are connected to inflammation in our organs, including our brains, and thus impacts the processes for aging and sense of balance and well-being. In addition, social isolation and loneliness can impact risk for depression, cognitive decline, and risk for AD/ADRD. More research is needed to understand how social and environmental determinants impact healthy aging and the role of nutrition and the microbiome on preventing and mediating the risk for dementia.

As research progresses, including more diverse communities in biomedical and community-based research is an urgent imperative. Clinical trials conducted to date have failed to achieve meaningful representation by minoritized and low-income communities, leading to results that are not generalizable to many of the Americans in greatest need of these therapies. Reducing health disparities among older people is critical to slowing or reversing the physical impacts of AD/ADRD and improving the health of older people overall. Toward that end, financial resources and community-engaged strategies are needed to ensure that the promise of biomedical research and clinical trials is available to all. Population health approaches offer ways to work hand-in-hand with diverse communities to address a range of aging-related conditions, including AD/ADRD, and are critical to informing the development of primary and secondary prevention strategies that aim to increase health equity for all Americans.

These challenges are daunting – but not insurmountable. This Handbook aims to provide a starting point for clinicians and other practitioners eager to take on these challenges in innovative, meaningful ways, particularly in minoritized, limited English proficient, and low-income communities. The topics included here range from population health trends and approaches to understanding community and patient engagement to caregiver perspectives and emerging trends. The Handbook aims to serve as a primer, introducing fundamental aspects of population health and participatory approaches to reducing health disparities and advancing health equity in the context of aging-related research. Our hope is that this introduction to the landscape of aging research in the most vulnerable of our communities will facilitate creativity, compassion, and meaningful next steps in biomedical and socioecological research, community support, and clinical care.

Chau Trinh-Shevrin, DrPH
Professor, Departments of Population Health and Medicine,
NYU Grossman School of Medicine

REFERENCES

Ackley, S. F., Zimmerman, S. C., Brenowitz, W. D., Tchetgen Tchetgen, E. J., Gold, A. L., Manly, J. J., Mayeda, E. R., Filshtein, T. J., Power, M. C., Elahi, F. M., Brickman, A. M., & Glymour, M. M. (2021). Effect of reductions in amyloid levels on cognitive change in randomized trials: Instrumental variable meta-analysis. *BMJ (Clinical Research Ed.)*, 372, n156. https://doi.org/10.1136/bmj.n156

THE EDITOR

CHAU TRINH-SHEVRIN, DrPH is Professor in the Departments of Population Health and Medicine, Vice Chair for Research, Director of the Section for Health Equity, and Institutional Review Board Chair at NYU Grossman School of Medicine. For over 25 years, her research focuses on the rigorous development and evaluation of multilevel strategies to reduce health disparities and advance health equity among low-income and across diverse racial and ethnic groups.

Dr. Trinh-Shevrin is multi-principal investigator (MPI) of a National Institute on Minority Health and Health Disparities (NIMHD) Center of Excellence, the NYU Center for the Study of Asian American Health (CSAAH), and a National Institute on Aging (NIA) Engagement in Longevity and Medicine Research Collaborative. Dr. Trinh-Shevrin also led a Centers for Disease Control and Prevention (CDC) Research Center for over a decade and currently leads a CDC Cancer Prevention and Control Research Network Center. Building on her expertise in community-based participatory research and longstanding relationships with national and local community partners, she is MPI of a National Institutes of Health (NIH) Community Engagement Alliance to End COVID-19 Disparities and associate director of Community Outreach and Engagement for the Perlmutter Cancer Center, a National Cancer Institute-designated Comprehensive Cancer Center.

Dr. Trinh-Shevrin is dedicated to mentoring junior faculty and students in minority and health disparities research. She is involved in many NIH-funded research training and education programs and leads an NIA Academic Leadership Award to support mentored research opportunities in healthy aging and health disparities research.

Dr. Trinh-Shevrin earned her doctorate in public health from the Mailman School of Public Health, Columbia University, and masters in health policy and management at the State University of New York at Albany. She has coauthored more than 150 peer-reviewed publications and is coeditor of three textbooks, *Applied Population Health Approaches for Asian American Communities* (Jossey-Bass, 2023), *Asian American Communities and Health* (Jossey-Bass, 2009), and *Empowerment and Recovery: Confronting Addiction during Pregnancy with Peer Counseling* (Praeger Press, 1998).

THE CONTRIBUTORS

JEANNETTE MICHELE BEASLEY, PhD, MPH, RDN, is an Assistant Professor in the Departments of Nutrition and Food Studies and Medicine at NYU. She trained in biology at the College of William and Mary (BS), nutrition at University of North Carolina-Chapel Hill (MPH, RDN) and epidemiology at the Johns Hopkins Bloomberg School of Public Health (PhD). Her research focuses on understanding the role of nutrition in chronic disease prevention, particularly in furthering the understanding of the role of nutrition in the prevention of cardiovascular disease in diverse populations and refining recommendations regarding the protein needs of older adults. This work has resulted in over 75 peer-reviewed publications and 8 books or book chapters. She has received funding from National Institutes of Health, Centers for Disease Control, and private foundations. She serves as an Associate Editor for BMC Public Health and as a peer reviewer for over 20 other academic journals. She previously held academic appointments at Group Health Research Institute, Fred Hutchinson Cancer Research Center, and Albert Einstein College of Medicine.

ABRAHAM AIZER BRODY, PhD, RN, FAAN, is the Mathy Mezey Professor of Geriatric Nursing, Professor of Medicine, and Associate Director of the Hartford Institute for Geriatric Nursing at NYU. His work focuses on the intersection of geriatrics, palliative care, quality, and equity. The primary goal of his research, clinical, and policy pursuits is to improve the quality of care for older adults with serious illnesses wherever they reside through the development, testing, and dissemination of real-world, technology, and informatics-supported quality improvement interventions. He is the principal investigator of multiple large-scale pragmatic clinical trials to improve the quality of care and quality of life for persons living with dementia and their care partners living in the community, and leads the Pilot Core for the National Institute on Aging (NIA) IMPACT Collaboratory, which is a collaboration with NIA to move evidence-based practices for persons living with dementia from research to practice. He maintains an active practice on the geriatrics and palliative care consult services at NYU Langone Health.

OMONIGHO MICHAEL BUBU, MD, PhD, MPH, is an Assistant Professor and physician scientist at NYU Grossman School of Medicine, in the Departments of Psychiatry and Population Health, with a programmatic research focus on sleep, aging, and Alzheimer's disease (AD). Dr. Bubu has graduate, internship, and fellowship-level clinical and research training in neurology, neuro-epidemiology, and public health. His research examines how age-related and age-dependent sleep changes, and vascular risk, impact cognitive decline and AD risk, and how they drive AD-related disparities.

MIRNOVA E. CEÏDE, MD, MSc, is an Assistant Professor of Geriatric Psychiatry and Geriatrics at the Albert Einstein College of Medicine/Montefiore Medical Center, the Assistant Program Director of the Montefiore Geriatric Psychiatry Fellowship, and Associate Director of Psychiatry at the Montefiore Center for the Aging Brain. She completed her Geriatric Psychiatry Fellowship at SUNY Downstate and joined the Geriatric Psychiatry Division at Montefiore Medical Center in 2013. She has presented at national and international meetings on behavioral risk factors for dementia and models of psychiatric integration in health care. In 2018, she completed the Albert Einstein Clinical Research Training Program and attained a Master of Science in Clinical Research. She completed a Columbia Center for Interdisciplinary Research on Alzheimer's disease Disparities (CIRAD) Pilot Project Grant to further apathy and cognition in a racially and ethnically diverse clinic population. Most recently, she was awarded a National Institutes of Health Diversity Supplement to study apathy as an early risk factor for dementia in a multicountry cohort of older adults.

RUIJIA CHEN, ScD, is a social epidemiologist and a postdoctoral scholar in the Department of Epidemiology and Biostatistics at the University of California, San Francisco. She received her Doctor of Science degree in social epidemiology from Harvard University and master's degree in social policy from the University of Pennsylvania. Her research focuses on applying advanced epidemiologic methods to understand how psychosocial determinants across the life course influence social disparities in late-life cognitive outcomes.

JOSHUA CHODOSH, MD, MSHS, is Director of the NYU Division of Geriatric Medicine and Palliative Care and the inaugural endowed Michael L. Freedman Professor of Geriatric Research at NYU Grossman School of Medicine. He is also Staff Physician at VA NY Harbor Healthcare System. As Professor of Medicine and Population Health, Dr. Chodosh joined NYU in 2015 after a productive research career at UCLA and the Greater Los Angeles VA. At NYU, he has built the Freedman Research Center on Aging, Technology and Cognitive Health supported by investigators that cross several departments including medicine, population health, surgery, and emergency medicine and multiple institutions across the United States. Dr. Chodosh is PI or MPI of multiple National Institutes of Health R01s and a VA multisite Merit. He is also PI of the Centers for Disease Control and Prevention BOLD Public Health Center of Excellence on Early Detection of Dementia and leads the Outreach, Recruitment, and Engagement Core of the NYU Alzheimer's Disease Research Center. In 2017, Dr. Chodosh cofounded the NYU Aging Incubator, a University-wide, educational, and research collective serving the larger University community.

■ ■ ■

OHSHUE GATANAGA, MPH(c), MSSW(c), is currently a graduate student studying social work and public health at Columbia University. His research focuses on infusing syndemics and intersectionality theories to examine how multiple marginalized identities impact behavioral health and substance use outcomes. In particular, Gatanaga is interested in exploring historically under-researched communities, such as Asian American subgroups and LGBTQ+ communities. Other current and related research projects include partnering on National Institutes of Health grants addressing intersectional stigma among men who have sex with men, the HIV/AIDS intervention BRIDGE (Improving HIV Service Delivery for People who Inject Drugs in Kazakhstan), and gender-based violence studies for Project E-Worth (Multimedia HIV/STI Intervention for Black Drug-Involved women on Probation in New York City). As an aspiring practitioner-scholar, Gatanaga hopes to conduct research at the forefront of clinical implementation. He is currently a member of the New York State Society for Clinical Social Work, the American Public Health Association LGBTQ Health Caucus, and the American Public Health Association Asian and Pacific Islander Caucus for Public Health.

■ ■ ■

NISHA GODBOLE, BS, is a third-year medical student at Stony Brook University in New York. She became interested early during her medical education on Aging and Alzheimer's disease and related dementias. She pursued funded research through the NYU Grossman School of Medicine, Department of Medicine and Engagement and Longevity in Medicine (ELM) research collaborative.

■ ■ ■

LU HU, PhD, is a behavioral scientist and an Assistant Professor in the Department of Population Health at NYU Langone Health. Her research primarily focuses on developing and testing innovative, sustainable, and scalable technology-based interventions to increase access to care and reduce health disparities in underserved populations with chronic conditions.

■ ■ ■

TERRY T-K HUANG, PhD, MPH, MBA, is Professor and Chair of the Department of Health Policy and Management, Director of the Center for Systems and Community Design, and Co-Director of the NYU-CUNY Prevention Research Center (Centers for Disease Control and Prevention-designated) at the City University of New York Graduate School of Public Health and Health Policy (CUNY SPH). In addition to his academic research endeavors, Dr. Huang founded a public health entrepreneurship platform, Firefly Innovations (www.firefly-innovations.com), at the CUNY SPH and leads a new angel portfolio fund, COREangels Health Equity & Mental Wellbeing. He received the United States Department of Health and Human Services Secretary's Innovation Award in 2010 and the National Institutes of Health Director's Award in 2011. In addition, he received the National Cancer Institute Award of Merit in 2012. Dr. Huang holds a PhD in Preventive Medicine and an MPH from the University of Southern California, an MBA from IE Business School (Madrid, Spain), and a BA in Psychology from McGill University (Montreal, Canada).

JAY M. IYER, AB(c), is a sophomore at Harvard College concentrating in Molecular and Cellular Biology and Statistics. He is a researcher in the Department of Stem Cell and Regenerative Biology at Harvard University, investigating the potentially selective distribution of specific ribosomal proteins in neuronal subtypes and their respective subcellular compartments. Furthermore, he is a researcher in the Department of Neurology at Massachusetts General Hospital, where he analyzes data from clinical cohorts to discover predictors of Parkinson's Disease and Progressive Supranuclear Palsy (PSP) progression. Iyer also leads his nonprofit organization, MIND Relief, which provides support to patients and families with rare neurodegenerative diseases such as PSP. He further serves as the director of Harvard College Alzheimer's Buddies, where he assists individuals with Alzheimer's disease and related dementias.

KALISHA BONDS JOHNSON, PhD, RN, PMHNP-BC, is an Assistant Professor at Emory University's Nell Hodgson Woodruff School of Nursing in Atlanta, Georgia and a Psychiatric Mental Health Nurse Practitioner at Emory University's Integrated Memory Care, a primary care clinic tailored to the care of persons living with dementia. She graduated from The University of Tennessee at Martin with a Bachelor of Science in Nursing in 2007. In 2012, she graduated with a Master of Science in Nursing from Vanderbilt University, specializing as a Family Psychiatric Mental Health Nurse Practitioner. In 2019, Dr. Bonds Johnson graduated with a PhD from Oregon Health & Science University. Most recently, she completed her postdoctoral training at Emory University from 2019 to 2021. Dr. Bonds Johnson's research focuses on improving the quality of life of African American persons living with dementia and their family care partners. Specifically, this research focuses on the creation of culturally tailored interventions to improve the decision-making processes of adult daughters navigating the health care system for a parent living with dementia while considering individual, family, community, and societal factors.

LISA A. JUCKETT, PhD, OTR/L, is an Assistant Professor of Occupational Therapy at The Ohio State University. Her research centers on bridging the gap between empirical discoveries and the use of these discoveries in real-world practice settings. Heavily informed by the field of implementation science, Dr. Juckett's research examines the factors and strategies that influence evidence-based practice uptake, primarily in organizations that serve the older adult population. Specifically, Dr. Juckett's work aims to develop and test implementation strategies that support the use of evidence-based practices in the contexts of (a) stroke rehabilitation and (b) home- and community-based service systems. Active involvement of community and clinical partners is a hallmark characteristic of Dr. Juckett's research, resulting in several collaborations with entities that provide immensely valuable health and human services to the older adult community.

■ ■ ■

AISHA T. LANGFORD, PhD, MPH, is an Assistant Professor in the Department of Population Health NYU Grossman School of Medicine. Under NYU Langone Health's Clinical and Translational Science Institute, she co-directs the Recruitment and Retention Core (RRC). In her role as RRC co-director, Dr. Langford advises study teams across the medical school on recruitment feasibility and ways to maximize participant retention, covering all stages of clinical trial and health research study design. A large proportion of these consultations include ways to enhance inclusion of women, racial/ethnic minorities, and adults aged 65 and older in clinical research. Dr. Langford advocates that researchers should ensure that all eligible patients are invited to participate in clinical trials and that underrepresented populations in research have equitable access to research opportunities, which often means addressing the logistical and communication barriers that may hinder participation. Dr. Langford earned her BA in English from the University of Virginia, MPH in Behavioral Science from Saint Louis University, and PhD in Health Behavior and Health Education from the University of Michigan.

■ ■ ■

MATTHEW LEE, DrPH, MPH, is an Assistant Professor in the Section for Health Equity and the Center for the Study of Asian American Health within the Department of Population Health at NYU Grossman School of Medicine. Dr. Lee earned their doctorate in Sociomedical Sciences from the Columbia University Mailman School of Public Health and was also a Robert Wood Johnson Foundation Health Policy Research Scholar. As a community-engaged implementation scientist and critical health equity researcher, Dr. Lee's research applies participatory approaches and mixed methods to examine the reach and impact of policies and evidence-based interventions within structurally underserved communities. Broadly, Dr. Lee is focused on improving the equitable implementation and sustainability of policies and programs to eliminate health disparities and advance health justice.

■ ■ ■

SAHNAH LIM, PhD, MPH, MIA, is an Assistant Professor who is leading the Gender Equity scientific track and Mental Health scientific track at NYU Grossman School of Medicine's Department of Population Health's Section for Health Equity. As a health equity researcher, Dr. Lim conducts applied, community-engaged studies that seek to address gender-related health issues among hard-to-reach populations such as sex workers and immigrant survivors of gender-based violence. Her research uses intersectionality and syndemics frameworks to understand how multiple marginalization impacts mental and sexual health outcomes.

■ ■ ■

DAVID W. LOUNSBURY, PhD, is Associate Professor in the Department of Epidemiology & Population Health and Associate Director of Patient-Centered Outcomes Research Training at the Albert Einstein College of Medicine, New York, USA. His domestic and international research is directed toward implementation of evidence-based, community-facing health services for prevention and treatment of chronic health conditions (cancer, diabetes/obesity, HIV/AIDS, opioid use disorder, depression, and dementia) in medically underserved populations. He applies ecologically grounded social science methodologies, such as action research and system dynamics modeling, as a means of participatory problem-solving to address complex multilevel problems in health care delivery. Dr. Lounsbury is also a Faculty Fellow with the Center for Systems & Community Design (City University of New York, Graduate School of Public Health & Health Policy) and currently serves as Co-Chair of the System Dynamics Society's Psychology and Human Behavior Special Interest Group.

■ ■ ■

DEBORAH K. MIN, MPH, is a Senior Project Coordinator at the NYU Center for the Study of Asian American Health (CSAAH) based in the Department of Population Health's Section for Health Equity at NYU Grossman School of Medicine. She is also a doctoral candidate at the Johns Hopkins Bloomberg School of Public Health within the Health Equity and Social Justice track. Her research interests include community-driven and culturally tailored projects that confront health disparities and advance health equity within and across Asian American communities. She received her BA in Psychology at Wheaton College (IL) and MPH from Columbia University's Mailman School of Public Health, Department of Sociomedical Sciences with a concentration in Child, Youth, and Family Health.

■ ■ ■

SUPRIYA MISRA, ScD, is currently an Assistant Professor in the Department of Public Health at San Francisco State University and a Faculty Scholar in the Health Equity Institute at San Francisco State University. Her research focuses on mental health inequities among socially marginalized communities, particularly racial and ethnic minority groups. She uses mixed methods to understand the roles of racism, stigma, and trauma on the onset and experience of mental distress and to promote dignity and justice for those living with mental illness. Dr. Misra completed her BA and MA in Psychology at Stanford University, her ScD in Social and Behavioral Sciences at the Harvard T.H. Chan School of Public Health, and a Provost's Postdoctoral Fellowship at NYU. She also worked for several years in nonprofit management to develop and implement evidence-based health education resources.

■ ■ ■

KOMAL PATEL MURALI, PhD, RN, ACNP-BC, is an Assistant Professor at NYU Rory Meyers College of Nursing. Her primary program of research focuses on improving end-of-life and hospice care transitions for seriously ill persons living with dementia in the home health care setting. Additionally, Dr. Murali aims to develop care coordination interventions to facilitate equitable hospice use among racially and ethnically diverse persons living with dementia. As a nurse scientist and board-certified acute care nurse practitioner with a background in critical care, Dr. Murali is also passionate about end-of-life decision making and palliative care integration in the intensive care unit.

BETH PRUSACZYK, MSW, PhD, is an Assistant Professor at the Institute for Informatics and in General Medical Sciences at Washington University School of Medicine in St. Louis. Her research focuses on improving health care and social services for older adults living in rural areas, especially vulnerable older adults such as those with dementia or low income, by understanding how to better implement existing research findings into practice and policy. Her work also focuses on how network science and health information technology can both inform and speed this implementation process. Dr. Prusaczyk received her PhD and MSW from the Brown School of Social Work at Washington University in St. Louis and completed her postdoctoral training at Vanderbilt University Medical Center. She also served as a 2018–2019 Health and Aging Policy Fellow, working in the United States Senate on the Special Committee on Aging. She has her undergraduate degree in journalism from Webster University and worked as a journalist prior to her career in research.

STUART F. QUAN, MD, is a Senior Physician in the Division of Sleep and Circadian Disorders at Brigham and Women's Hospital and the Gerald E. McGinnis Professor of Sleep Medicine at Harvard Medical School. In addition, he is Professor Emeritus of Medicine at the University of Arizona where he was Chief of Pulmonary and Critical Care Medicine, Associate Head of the Department of Medicine, Program Director of the GCRC, and Director of the Sleep Disorders Center. He also is an adjunct faculty member in the Arizona State University College of Nursing and Health Innovation. Dr. Quan is the Field Editor of Frontiers in Sleep, was the founding editor of the Journal of Clinical Sleep Medicine, and has served as President of the American Academy of Sleep Medicine. His current research activities focus on the epidemiology of sleep and sleep and circadian disorders. He has written over 400 publications in scientific journals and books, and has authored a number of educational products for the general public.

REBECCA ROBBINS, MMSci, PhD, is an Instructor in Medicine at Harvard Medical School and an Associate Scientist at the Brigham and Women's Hospital. In her research, Dr. Robbins designs and evaluates novel interventions to improve sleep and sleep disorders among underserved communities. She has published more than 60 scientific articles. Dr. Robbins has held teaching positions at the Weill Cornell Medical College in Doha, Qatar and at Harvard College.

■ ■ ■

NASIM S. SABOUNCHI, PhD, MSc, is an Associate Professor at the City University of New York (CUNY) Graduate School of Public Health and Health Policy where she is also affiliated with the Center for Systems and Community Design (CSCD). She is an industrial and systems engineer, and a systems scientist in the field of public health and health care and recipient of the Systems Science Scholarship, Academy of Health – Robert Wood Johnson Foundation. Her research interest involves adopting tools including systems science methodologies, systems engineering and data analytics to model complex systems and problems pertaining to health outcomes at both the individual and population levels. Dr. Sabounchi contributes to the advancement of system dynamics modeling and computer simulation for studying complex health and social systems, and leads various projects in the domain of public health and health policy analysis including those that focus on the opioid epidemic, obesity, infectious disease, enhancing access to care for socio-economically disadvantaged populations, antibiotic resistance, Lyme Disease, and epidemics.

■ ■ ■

RACHEL SACKS, MPH, is an independent public health consultant specializing in scientific and technical writing. Prior to establishing her consulting business in 2006, she served in managerial positions with nonprofit organizations, a university-based research center, and a public health department in Bangkok, Thailand; Mumbai, India; and New York City, USA. She received her bachelor's degree at Tufts University in International Relations and French and her master's degree in public health at Yale University School of Medicine in the Division of International Health.

■ ■ ■

TINA R. SADARANGANI, PhD, RN, ANP-BC, GNP-BC, is a National Institutes of Health-funded Principal Investigator and board-certified primary care nurse practitioner. She is cross-appointed as an Assistant Professor at NYU Grossman School of Medicine's Department of Population Health. Her program of research is underscored by a profound commitment to advancing the health of minoritized older adults by leveraging the strengths of community-based adult day health care centers to target health disparities. In the last three years, she has expanded her program of research to focus on identifying and addressing the health care needs of cognitively impaired older immigrants, by using the adult day health center as a platform for the delivery of culturally and linguistically congruent care. Her on-going collaborations with the California Association of Adult Day Services, as well as other community-based organizations, have demonstrated that integrating adult day centers into the health care continuum contributes to reductions in avoidable health care utilization. Dr. Sadarangani's latest work focuses on improving communication between adult day centers and primary care providers using low-cost mobile technology. She recently received a K23 Career Development Award from the National Institute on Aging (NIA) as well as an R21 from NIA.

■ ■ ■

SCOTT E. SHERMAN, MD, MPH, is a Professor of Population Health, Medicine and Psychiatry at NYU Grossman School of Medicine. He received his MD from NYU School of Medicine and completed an MPH in Epidemiology/Biostatistics at Boston University School of Public Health. He is a practicing physician in internal medicine and geriatrics and sees patients at the Veterans Health Administration (VA) in New York. His research studies have focused on how to redesign health care systems to better help people quit smoking. Dr. Sherman is particularly focused on population health studies, examining the effectiveness of interventions in routine practice, as well as how to disseminate and implement them. He helped start and co-leads the NYU Clinical and Translational Science Institute Recruitment and Retention Core, which focuses on increasing recruitment into federal research, particularly recruiting groups that are underrepresented in clinical research. Dr. Sherman has over 225 peer-reviewed publications in scientific journals and is currently leading 7 large grants, with funding from the National Institutes of Health, the VA, and foundations.

■ ■ ■

RACHEL L. THOMPSON, MS, is a PhD student studying Environmental and Planetary Health Sciences at the City University of New York (CUNY) Graduate School of Public Health and Health Policy (New York, NY) where she also works as a research associate at the CUNY Center for Systems and Community Design (CSCD). Thompson holds a Master of Science degree from Grand Valley State University (Grand Rapids, MI) in biostatistics and has several years of experience in public health and basic sciences research. Over the course of her academic and professional career, she has contributed to a variety of research projects spanning a range of public health and health policy domains, including social determinants of health, substance use, environmental health, and infectious disease. Thompson's research interests center on using system dynamics and geospatial modeling techniques to study complex health and socio-ecological systems. Her current research contributes to National Institutes of Health-funded projects using group model building and system dynamics modeling to design and evaluate evidence-based practices for opioid overdose prevention and treatment for opioid use disorder.

■ ■ ■

BEI WU, PhD, is Vice Dean for Research and Dean's Professor in Global Health at the NYU Rory Meyers College of Nursing. Dr. Wu is currently leading several National Institutes of Health-funded projects including a clinical trial to improve oral health for persons with cognitive impairment. She co-leads the Rutgers-NYU Center for Asian Health Promotion and Equity. Through this center, she leads a 5-year intervention study that focuses on supporting Chinese and Korean dementia caregivers. Dr. Wu is a Principal Investigator of the National Institute on Aging-funded Asian Resource Center for Minority Aging. Her extensive publications cover a wide range of areas on aging and health, with a particular focus on risk factors related to cognitive impairment, dementia caregiving, and geriatric oral health. Dr. Wu is a fellow of the Gerontological Society of America and the New York Academy of Medicine. She is also an Honorary Fellow of the American Academy of Nursing.

JIAQI YANG, BS, currently is a master's student at the Johns Hopkins Bloomberg School of Public Health, pursuing a degree in Cardiovascular and Clinical Epidemiology. She received her bachelor's degree in Nutrition and Dietetics at NYU. Yang's research mainly examines how healthy dietary patterns influence chronic disease risk, particularly focusing on cardiovascular disease and cognitive decline in elderly populations.

ACKNOWLEDGMENTS

This book was supported in part by the National Institute on Aging (NIA) Award Number K07AG068186, the National Institutes of Health (NIH) National Institute on Minority Health and Health Disparities (NIMHD) Award Number U54MD000538, and the Centers for Disease Control and Prevention (CDC) Award Number CDC NU58DP006911. The content is solely the responsibility of the authors and does not necessarily represent the official views of the NIA, NIMHD, or CDC.

CHAPTER

OVERVIEW OF POPULATION TRENDS IN AGING AND ALZHEIMER'S DISEASE AND ALZHEIMER'S DISEASE-RELATED DEMENTIA (AD/ADRD) DISPARITIES

CHAU TRINH-SHEVRIN, TINA R. SADARANGANI, RACHEL SACKS, DEBORAH K. MIN

LEARNING OBJECTIVES

By the end of this chapter, readers will be able to:

- Describe demographic changes occurring among the United States (US) population as a whole and among the subpopulation of older adults.
- Articulate ways in which health disparities uniquely impact racial and ethnic minoritized, low income, and other vulnerable older adults.
- Identify key health issues affecting older adults in the US.

Population Science Methods and Approaches to Aging and Alzheimer's Disease and Related Dementias Research, First Edition. Edited by Chau Trinh-Shevrin.
© 2024 John Wiley & Sons, Inc. Published 2024 by John Wiley & Sons, Inc.

INTRODUCTION

This chapter describes demographic trends and health issues impacting the health of older people in the United States (US) and identifies unique challenges and concerns related to healthy aging among racial and ethnic minoritized populations, including disproportionate incidence of Alzheimer's disease and Alzheimer's disease-related dementias (AD/ADRD). As the aging population becomes more diverse, the National Institute on Aging (National Institute on Aging, 2019) and the US Department of Health and Human Services have called for strategies that focus on improving the health of older people in diverse populations and specifically improving health outcomes for racial and ethnic minoritized populations by addressing factors that underpin disparities, such as access to care (United States Department of Health and Human Services, 2019). Summarizing these issues in a concise manner is difficult because of manifold demographic, cultural, and societal changes impacting the rapidly growing and diversifying population of older Americans. This chapter aims to present an overview and introduction to this shifting landscape, offering a foundation upon which more detailed discussions of these various issues will be constructed in the chapters that follow.

DEMOGRAPHIC TRENDS

As a whole, the US population is growing older (US Census Bureau, 2020). Longer lifespans and aging baby boomers – that is, the generation born between 1946 and 1964 – are the two key drivers of this growth contributing to an increase in the national median age from 37.2 years in 2010 to 38.4 years in 2019. Regional differences in the aging population are notable, with over half of states having a median age older than 38.4 years, including all 9 states of the Northeast region, 11 states in the South, 6 in the Midwest, and 3 in the West. In Maine, Florida, West Virginia, and Vermont, one in five people were aged 65 or older in 2019. It is estimated that by 2030, older adults will comprise 20% of the US population overall, representing an increase of 22% from 2014 (Matthews et al., 2019).

Importantly, racial and ethnic minoritized populations are aging at a faster rate than the non-Hispanic White (White) population (CDC, 2020). In 2020, only 10% of racial and ethnic minoritized groups were aged 65 or older, whereas 21% of non-Hispanic White (White) people were older adults (Administration for Community Living, 2022). Of the total population of older Americans (aged 65 or older), 77% was White alone, 9% was Black (Black) alone, 5% was Asian American alone, 0.6% was American Indian or Alaska Native (AI/AN), and 0.1% was Native Hawaiian or Pacific Islander (NH/PI). Eight percent identified as Hispanic (Latine) of any race and 6% as two or more racial or ethnic groups (ACL, 2022). In contrast to these relatively small proportions, some estimates predict that by 2060, among people aged 65 or older, racial and ethnic minoritized adults will represent 45% of the population (Matthews et al., 2019). The Latine population is expected to increase by 391%, the AI/AN population by 274%, the combined Asian American and NH/PI populations by 270%, and the Black population by 172%. In comparison, the White population is predicted to increase by only 75%.

As the US population ages and diversifies, the health care system will face growing challenges related to paying for and delivering care to older Americans. Overall, health care spending is projected to increase by 25% by 2030, from $555 billion to $903 billion (CDC,

2013). A disproportionate amount of this spending will be among older Americans with expanding health care needs, particularly in the last few weeks or months of life (Zayas et al., 2016). In parallel, poverty disproportionately impacts older Americans. In 2020, 9% of Americans age 65–74 lived in poverty compared with 14% of Americans age 85 and older (ACL, 2022). Poverty rates are impacted by race, ethnicity, and gender, with the lowest rates of poverty seen among White people and men age 65 and over. These trends signify an urgent need to introduce new frameworks to guide health care spending and refocus medical and social services toward older Americans experiencing the greatest health disparities. Tailoring services to a diverse range of population groups among older adults with unique linguistic, cultural, and logistical needs will be an essential premise of health care policy and program development in the decades ahead.

HEALTH INEQUITIES AMONG OLDER PEOPLE

Health inequities refer to disparities in health and health care that are associated with social, economic, and/or environmental disadvantage, resulting in disproportionate burdens of disease and disability among some groups of people as compared to others. Health inequities impact racial and ethnic minoritized populations as well as groups defined by immigrant status, disability, sex, gender, and geography. At the individual level, inequities in health and health care pose obstacles to overcoming social disadvantage, while at the population level, health inequities reinforce and compound the negative impacts of systemic injustice experienced by vulnerable groups (Braveman et al., 2011). Moreover, because systemic injustice is experienced across the life course, health inequities emerge among different population groups in utero and early life and become increasingly entrenched with increasing age. Thus, even as life expectancy and overall health have improved for most Americans, not all older adults have benefitted equally, with outcomes linked to race, gender, and economic status (CDC, 2013). Gaining a better understanding of the complex impacts of the biologic and social determinants of health (SDOH) on diverse racial and ethnic groups across the life course is essential to developing appropriate interventions and policy responses to ameliorate race-based health inequities among older adults. SDOH are defined as nonmedical factors impacting health and well-being, including the conditions in which people are born, grow, work, live, and age and the broader set of systems and forces that shape daily life (CDC, 2022a).

In all age groups, the overall health status of people of Latine, Asian American, Black, AI/AN, and NH/PI descent lags behind that of White people (CDC, 2013). Racial and ethnic minoritized older adults often experience the effects of health inequities more intensely than younger people for numerous reasons. Among older Black and Latine people, an increased risk for morbidity is often attributed to lower socioeconomic status (SES) and limited health care access among these populations (McGrath et al., 2019). However, limited English proficiency (LEP), differing cultural norms, and immigration status also impact health access, overall health status, and specific disease outcomes (CDC, 2013). Asian American and Latine communities are particularly affected by the intersection of social position, stigmatized immigrant stereotypes, and high rates of LEP. Adequate consideration of these factors demands more nuanced, multilayered approaches and disaggregated data collection to support the development of effective health promotion strategies and interventions among an increasingly diverse older population.

Immigration status is a particularly complex and understudied factor (Moon et al., 2019). Typically, data show that immigrants are initially healthier than the US-born population but that over time, risk profiles for foreign- and US-born populations become more similar due to acculturation and other factors; and in older age groups, immigrant populations may have poorer health status than US-born counterparts, as linguistic and other barriers limit foreign-born older adults' access to health care and health insurance (Bacong & Đoàn, 2022). Among older immigrant adults, systemic racism and social disadvantage may exert an even stronger impact on health status than among younger immigrant adults. As an example, higher AD/ADRD prevalence has been documented among older immigrant White and Latine people as compared to US-born counterparts, while foreign-born Black people have lower rates of AD/ADRD than US-born Blacks (Moon et al., 2019). One potential explanation for these differences is that US-born Black people endure the persistent negative and intergenerational effects of systemic racism on their health across the entire life course within the specific context of the history and legacies of slavery, segregation, and White Supremacy in the US. In contrast, foreign-born Black people may have different life experiences with systemic and interpersonal racism in their countries of origin and may be impacted by historical and contemporary racism and colorism differently across generations. Yet this phenomenon of risk based on nativity remains poorly understood.

Meanwhile, despite being the fastest growing and most ethnically diverse immigrant population in the US, Asian American people have been understudied and historically disinvested in research funding (Đoàn et al., 2019). "Asian American" refers to individuals with origins in East Asia, South Asia, or Southeast Asia and includes more than 20 ethnic groups with differing languages, geographic origins, immigration histories, and acculturation status (Budiman & Ruiz, 2021). One California-based study found differences in dementia risk across Asian ethnic groups, underscoring the need for data disaggregated by ethnic group and for future research to elucidate the role of immigration status, acculturation, and SES within and across Asian groups on dementia prevalence and risk (Mayeda et al., 2017). The lack of data describing Asian immigrants has posed a significant obstacle to understanding the role of systemic racism and discrimination on their health (Gee et al., 2009). The effects of discrimination and systemic racism on health status are further discussed in Chapter 3.

More broadly, the disproportionate prevalence of chronic health conditions among older racialized and minoritized people as compared to older White people provides a key example of the ways in which inequities may worsen among older Americans. Returning to the example of AD/ADRD, despite some evidence of racial differences in the impact of genetic factors by race, genetics do not account for the large differences in AD/ADRD prevalence or incidence among racial groups (Alzheimer's Association, 2021). Rather, health and SES disparities are linked to these outcomes through systemic factors rooted in discrimination and racism. Cardiovascular disease and diabetes, conditions with disproportionate prevalence among Black, Latine, Asian American, NH/PI, and AI/AN populations, are linked to AD/ADRD in older age groups overall and specifically to the higher AD/ADRD prevalence seen among older adults. These chronic conditions are associated with long-term exposure to adverse social and economic conditions, including living, working, learning, and playing in environments with limited access to nutritious foods, parks and other recreational spaces, clean air and water, safe housing, quality education, employment that guarantees a living wage, and other factors (Williams & Collins, 2001).

Perceptions of aging and healthy aging also differ among racial and ethnic groups, potentially impacting disparate health outcomes among various populations. One Los Angeles-based study found that Korean and Chinese American older adults had lower age-expectations than Black or Latine Americans – a finding that researchers suggested may be adaptive and, therefore, protective, for future well-being (Menkin et al., 2017). Black people had the highest age-expectations of these groups, a finding that may be explained in part by more positive perceptions of aging in individualistic societies, but may also contribute to poorer outcomes in older adults due to unrealistically high expectations of aging. Developing a better understanding of age expectations for these different populations could inform culturally appropriate clinical and community interventions for these groups.

Innovative study design, public health surveillance systems, patient and community engagement strategies, and analytic methods are needed that will allow for: 1) better assessment of health and social risk factors that emerge in childhood, early adulthood, and middle life and impact health inequities among diverse populations of older adults and 2) prevention and management of diseases that disproportionately impact different racial and ethnic minoritized groups. New approaches to developing such methodologies and strategies are discussed in Chapters 5, 6, and 7, respectively.

KEY HEALTH ISSUES IMPACTING OLDER ADULTS

Multimorbidity/Comorbidity

Multimorbidity, also referred to as comorbidity and defined as two or more co-occurring chronic illnesses, is endemic among older adults and is on the rise due to the combination of declining mortality rates and the aging of the population (Forman et al., 2018; Quiñones et al., 2019; Salive, 2013). Not surprisingly, multimorbidity is most common among those of most advanced age. More than 80% of adults age 80 and older have two or more chronic conditions, while 54% of adults age 85 and older have four or more conditions (Forman et al., 2018). The most common multimorbid conditions include cardiovascular, respiratory, and metabolic conditions – all of which have been shown to be individual risk factors for additional chronic illnesses, including dementia (Goodman et al., 2016). Notably, these common multimorbid conditions are associated with the five leading causes of death among all Americans age 65 and over – i.e., heart disease, cancer, respiratory conditions, stroke, and Alzheimer's disease (CDC, 2021b).

Multimorbidity often begins in younger age groups and is linked to various demographic factors including gender, education, marital status, income, and place of residence (Goodman et al., 2016). Longer, cumulative exposure to environmental, social, and biologic risk factors for the common diseases that comprise multimorbidity disproportionately impact Black people, Latine people, and other minoritized groups. These risk factors also disproportionately impact people with lower educational attainment and SES who have limited access to quality health care – groups that often overlap with racialized populations (Quiñones et al, 2019). In cases of chronic illnesses such as diabetes and hypertension, the health disparities that are pronounced in middle and older age groups could be reduced with better prevention and management of these conditions earlier in the life course (Beydoun et al., 2016; CDC, 2009; Wray et al., 2005). However, numerous barriers pose significant obstacles to improving outcomes in early adulthood for health disparity populations. These barriers include poor health care access (Bailey et al., 2017), a lack of health care workforce participation by minority communities (including LEP communities; Stanford, 2020), and lack of culturally tailored interventions for diverse groups (Joo & Liu, 2020). As a result, the health disparities gap continues to widen, leading to greater risk for multimorbidity disparities, poorer quality of life, and risk of AD/ADRD among older age groups. For this reason, a life course approach is critical to developing meaningful research to serve older adults from racial and ethnic minoritized populations.

AD/ADRD

AD is the most common cause of dementia and is the fifth leading cause of death among all adults 65 years or older (Alzheimer's Association, 2021). Prevalence of AD/ADRD has been estimated at 11% of US adults over 65 overall (Hebert et al., 2013) and by 2060, 13.9 million Americans are projected to have the disease (Matthews et al., 2019). As longevity increases globally, AD/ADRD is the key threat to well-being among people over 65, comprising the greatest challenge for health and social care in the 21st century (Livingston et al., 2017). Dementia impacts: 1) individuals with the condition, who progressively lose their memory, functional abilities, and independence; 2) their families and care partners or caregivers, who must cope with the decline and respond to the practical, health-related, and emotional needs of the affected individual; and 3) wider society, which must provide health and social care for the individuals and their families and caregivers. In terms of economic impact, nearly 85% of costs associated with AD/ADRD are related to family and social care, rather than medical treatment, highlighting the need for a systems-based approach to managing the disease and long-term care as well as indirect and direct costs of caregiving for individuals with AD/ADRD (Livingston et al., 2017).

One-third of dementia risk may be tied to modifiable environmental factors (Livingston et al., 2017), a finding that underscores the importance of developing tailored research among diverse population groups to explore the social determinants of AD/ADRD across the life course. For example, as compared to White people, research suggests that AD/ADRD prevalence among Black people is approximately double while prevalence among Latine people is about one and a half times (Alzheimer's Association, 2021). AI/AN older people are also more likely than White or Asian American people to develop AD/ADRD, with one in three AI/AN older individuals impacted by dementia (Alzheimer's Association, n.d.). Differences in prevalence of a variety of risk factors related to health, lifestyle, and SES among these disparate racial and ethnic groups likely contribute to these disparate rates of disease. In terms of health-related factors, cardiometabolic conditions that impact blood flow to the brain have also been linked to higher prevalence of AD. Strategies to prevent and manage these conditions in early and middle life, including the development and implementation of systemic interventions to provide support for healthier lifestyles overall, are critical to prevention and management of dementia in older age, particularly given that no disease-modifying treatments are available for dementia itself (Barthold et al., 2020). Yet studies show that people from racial and ethnic minoritized communities with low SES or education levels are not diagnosed with AD/ADRD until they reach an advanced stage of disease and that they receive fewer formal services than their White counterparts, resulting in worse health outcomes (Chodosh et al., 2018; Kenning et al. 2017; Sadarangani et al., 2020). This research underscores the need for increased attention to developing strategies and interventions that are tailored to the unique genetic, biologic, environmental, and social conditions within which different populations age, including a systemic effort to incorporate AD/ADRD early assessment and intervention into primary health care for racial and ethnic minoritized and vulnerable populations. A more detailed discussion of the SDOH and their impact on the health of older Americans is presented in Chapters 2 and 3.

Mental Health

Depression, Anxiety, Suicide High rates of poor mental health have been reported in older members of several racial and ethnic minoritized groups (Office of the Surgeon General, 2001). Worsening mental health in older adults can be attributed in part to physical illnesses that emerge as people age (e.g., pain, cancer, neurologic disorders) as well as lack of social connection (Conjero et al., 2018). Poor self-rated mental health is especially pronounced among older immigrants, who report more stress during the life course and worse mental health than their non-immigrant counterparts. Nationally, the incidence of major depression has been found to be more frequent among Latine and Black people relative to White people (Dunlop et al., 2003). Black women report higher levels of depressive symptoms compared to White women throughout later life (Spence et al., 2011) and studies have found a higher prevalence of depressive symptoms among older people of Asian Indian, Filipino, NH/PI, and AI/AN descent relative to White people (Hooker et al., 2019; Office of the Surgeon General, 2001). Finally, although the rate of suicide typically declines as people age, older Asian Americans, particularly women, are at greater risk of suicide compared with their counterparts in other racial groups (Bartels et al., 2002; Yang & WonPat-Borja, 2007). Suicidal ideation has been found to be more frequent among older Asian American women with comorbid depression, anxiety, and substance use, as compared with White, Black, and Latina older women. Older Asian American women also have higher rates of completed suicide than their counterparts in other racial groups.

Social Isolation and Loneliness Social isolation and loneliness are two distinct, but often related, concepts that contribute to worsening mental health as adults age – especially among immigrant and lesbian, gay, bisexual, transgender, queer (or questioning), and other (LGBTQ+) people. Social isolation is defined as an objective lack of social contact with others (e.g., living alone). By contrast, loneliness is subjective: it is the reported feeling of being socially isolated and lonely (National Academies of Science, Engineering, and Medicine, 2020). A report from the National Academies of Sciences, Engineering, and Medicine (NASEM) stated that one in three adults aged 45 and older feel lonely, and one in four adults aged 65 and over are socially isolated (NASEM, 2020). Research is clear that social isolation among older adults is associated with a number of negative physical and mental health outcomes including mortality and dementia (Taylor et al., 2019), while loneliness is associated with higher rates of depression, anxiety, and suicide (CDC, 2021a).

Current research suggests that older immigrant and LGBTQ+ persons experience loneliness more often than other groups (NASEM, 2020). For example, social isolation among Latina/o/x immigrants is driven by language barriers, complex family dynamics, and new, immature relationships in their new country that lack history. LGBTQ+ persons experience more stigma and discrimination compared to their peers that drives higher rates of loneliness.

Food Insecurity/Nutrition

Food insecurity, defined as the lack of access to nutritious food for an active, healthy life, disproportionately affects older adults (Feeding America, 2016). Prior to 2020, more than 8% of older adults in the United States were food insecure overall (Feeding America, 2016), with Black and Latine adults over 65 being over three times more likely to experience food insecurity than White or Asian American older people, placing them at disproportionate risk for food insecurity. Nearly one in five Black older adults was food insecure, compared to one in 18 White older adults (Rabbitt et al., 2016). Among Asian American people, there is significant heterogeneity among ethnic subgroups and the likelihood of food insecurity increases with age (Becerra et al., 2018).

During the novel coronavirus disease 2019 (COVID-19) pandemic, food insecurity increased overall, with disproportionate effects on Black, Latine, AI/AN, Asian American, and NH/PI communities and those with LEP (Niles et al., 2021). Older adults with food insecurity are more likely to have multiple nutritional insufficiencies. This phenomenon is attributable both to the reliance of food-insecure individuals on inexpensive foods, which are high in calories but low in nutrient density, and older adults' reduced physical ability to extract nutrients from food. Nutritional insufficiencies, in turn, can contribute to chronic disease, such as type 2 diabetes mellitus (Fitzgerald et al., 2011), as well as premature functional decline. For example, in one study of older adults, those with food insecurity had similar functional limitations to adults who were 15 years older and food secure (Gundersen & Ziliak, 2015). Risk factors for malnutrition vary considerably according to racial group. In one study of adult day center participants, risk of malnutrition in Latine people was driven disproportionately by polypharmacy, by social isolation among Asian American people, and inadequate access to sufficient meals among Black people (Sadarangani et al., 2019a).

Novel Coronavirus Disease 2019 (COVID-19)

COVID-19, caused by severe acute respiratory syndrome coronavirus 2 (SARS-CoV-2), has killed over 1,000,000 people at the time of writing – 80% of whom are people over the age of 65 (CDC, 2022b). While COVID-19 is of particular concern for all older adults, those who are from racial and ethnic minoritized populations and those with LEP are at even greater risk of morbidity and mortality from this disease (CDC, 2022c). In addition to having higher cases and hospitalizations for COVID-19, Black and Latine individuals have nearly three times the death rate of White individuals (CDC, 2022c) and AI/AN and PI people are nearly twice as likely to die from COVID-19 as White people (CDC, 2020; Gawthrop, 2023).

While age, chronic conditions, and behavioral and social factors contribute to the severity of COVID-19 symptoms as well as the likelihood of mortality, the pandemic has also exposed the role of structural racism in shaping COVID-19 disparities and inequities in racial and ethnic minoritized populations (Ajilore & Thames, 2020). The "weathering" hypothesis suggests that increased exposure to social inequality throughout the life course results in physiological stress (Geronimus et al., 2006). Thus, COVID-19 has caused significant harm to older adults who are already vulnerable to poor health outcomes. Addressing structural factors underpinning inequities and designing and implementing successful vaccination campaigns that address vaccine hesitancy will be critical to reducing COVID-19 disparities impacting health inequities in older adults from communities of color.

During the initial vaccine rollout, the CDC showed similar vaccination rates between Latine and White people, and rates that exceeded White people among AI/AN, NH/PI, and Asian American people. However, the lowest rates of vaccination were found among Black individuals. Furthermore, Black and Latine Medicare beneficiaries had significantly lower rates of vaccination compared with White beneficiaries, particularly among those with an annual income under $25,000 per year (Cheng & Li, 2022). As of December 2022, uptake of the bivalent booster was higher among White people than all other racial and ethnic groups, excluding Asian Americans (CDC, 2022d). Age-adjusted COVID-19 infection rates illustrated the negative impact of these declining and disparate vaccination rates among diverse racial and ethnic groups. As of September 2022, age-adjusted COVID-19 infection rates were highest among Black and Latine people, followed by AI/AN people; while the lowest infection rates were found among White and Asian American and NH/PI people (Ndugga et al., 2022). Even among Asian American groups, subgroup data also demonstrated variation in vaccination rates and risk for COVID-related morbidity and mortality by ethnic group, with NH/PI people having significantly lower vaccination rates than Asian American people (Asian & Pacific Islander American Health Forum, 2021), underscoring the need for data disaggregated by ethnic group to understand the magnitude of risks within populations (Kalyanaraman et al., 2022).

CONCLUSION

As the US population ages and diversifies more rapidly than ever before, increased attention to the unique needs of racial and ethnic minoritized populations is imperative. Disparities persist across the life course, rendering older Americans from racial and ethnic minoritized backgrounds more vulnerable to debilitating health issues than their White counterparts and producing pronounced race- and ethnicity-based health inequities among older Americans. While multimorbidity, AD/ADRD, mental health issues, and COVID-19 disproportionately impact the older American population as a whole, extant data demonstrate the even greater impact of these conditions on racial and ethnic minoritized groups as compared to White people. More research is needed to understand how biologic factors and the SDOH impact the health status of racial and ethnic minoritized older adults.

In the chapters that follow, this handbook will introduce key topics related to aging and AD/ADRD research and propose strategies for integrating new methodologies to better understand and address issues impacting the health of older adults. Chapter 2 will introduce the SDOH and their impact on older adults, while Chapter 3 will explore the mechanisms through which systemic racism, stigma, and discrimination impact older adults, deepening health inequities among racial and ethnic minoritized and other vulnerable groups. Chapter 4 will address intersectionality, focusing on the unique issues that impact LGBTQ+ older adults who are members of racial and ethnic minoritized populations. Strategies for addressing these issues within aging research will then be explored. Chapter 5 will describe strategies for increasing the participation of older people in clinical research overall, Chapter 6 will introduce implementation science approaches to aging and AD/ADRD research and Chapter 7 will explore ways in which systems science methods may be applied to aging and AD/ADRD research. Chapter 8 will explore sleep and aging. Finally, Chapter 9 will present emerging research in the field of aging and AD/ADRD.

DISCUSSION QUESTIONS

1. Summarize some of the key demographic changes that the US population is undergoing and define what it means to have an aging population.

2. Discuss the ways in which health inequities impact among older adults. How might racially-based health inequities widen across the life course? How might inequities disproportionately impact older immigrants and other vulnerable subgroups?

3. Describe one health issue of concern for older adults. If you were researching this issue within one racial or ethnic minoritized group, what are some key questions you would pose? How might you tailor your study design to answer these questions?

REFERENCES

Administration for Community Living. (2022). 2021 Profile of older Americans. Available at: https://acl.gov/aging-and-disability-in-america/data-and-research/profile-older-americans. Accessed December 13, 2022.

Ajilore, O., & Thames, A. D. (2020). The fire this time: The stress of racism, inflammation and COVID-19. *Brain, Behavior, and Immunity, 88*, 66–67. https://doi.org/10.1016/j.bbi.2020.06.003

Alzheimer's Association. (2021). 2021 Alzheimer's disease facts and figures. *Alzheimer's & Dementia: The Journal of the Alzheimer's Association, 17*(3), 327–406. https://doi.org/10.1002/alz.12328

Alzheimer's Association. (n.d.). Native Americans and Alzheimer's. Available at: https://www.alz.org/help-support/resources/native-americans. Accessed December 13, 2022.

Asian & Pacific Islander Health Forum (APIAHF). (2021). Asian Americans, Native Hawaiians, and Pacific Islanders on COVID-19 and getting vaccinated. Available at: https://www.apiahf.org/resource/nationwide-survey-of-aanhpi-on-covid-19. Accessed December 20, 2022.

Bacong, A. M., & Đoàn, L. N. (2022). Immigration and the life course: Contextualizing and understanding health-care access and health of older adult immigrants. *Journal of Aging and Health, 34*(9–10), 1228–1243. https://doi.org/10.1177/08982643221104931

Bailey, Z. D., Krieger, N., Agénor, M., Graves, J., Linos, N., & Bassett, M. T. (2017). Structural racism and health inequities in the USA: Evidence and interventions. *Lancet, 389*, 1453–1463. https://doi.org/10.1016/S0140-6736(17)30569-X

Bartels, S. J., Coakley, E., Oxman, T. E., Constantino, G., Oslin, D., Chen, H., Zubritsky, C., Cheal, K., Durai, U. N., Gallo, J. J., Llorente, M., & Sanchez, H. (2002). Suicidal and death ideation in older primary care patients with depression, aniety, and at-risk alcohol use. *The American Journal of Geriatric Psychiatry: Official Journal of the American Association for Geriatric Psychiatry, 10*(4), 417–427. https://doi.org/10.1097/00019442-200207000-00008

Barthold, D., Joyce, G., Diaz Brinton, R., Wharton, W., Kehoe, P. G., & Zissimopoulos, J. (2020). Association of combination statin and antihypertensive therapy with reduced Alzheimer's disease and related dementia risk. *PloS One, 15*(3), e0229541. https://doi.org/10.1371/journal.pone.0229541

Becerra, M. B., Mshigeni, S. K., & Becerra, B. J. (2018). The overlooked burden of food insecurity among Asian Americans: Results from the California health interview survey. *International Journal of Environmental Research and Public Health, 15*(8), 1684. https://doi.org/10.3390/ijerph15081684

Beydoun, M. A., Beydoun, H. A., Mode, N., Dore, G. A., Caas, J. A., Eid, S. M., & Zonderman, A. B. (2016). Racial disparities in adult all-cause and cause-specific mortality among US adults: Mediating and moderating factors. *BMC Public Health, 16*(1), 1113. https://doi.org/10.1186/s12889-016-3744-z.

Braveman, P. A., Kumanyika, S., Fielding, J., Laveist, T., Borrell, L. N., Manderscheid, R., & Troutman, A. (2011). Health disparities and health equity: The issue is justice. *American Journal of Public Health, 101*(1), S149–S155. https://doi.org/10.2105/AJPH.2010.300062

Budiman, A., & Ruiz, N. G. (2021, April 29). *Key facts about Asian origin groups in the U.S.* Pew Research Center. Available at: https://www.pewresearch.org/fact-tank/2021/04/29/key-facts-about-asian-origin-groups-in-the-u-s Accessed December 3, 2022.

CDC. (2013). *The state of aging and health in the United States, 2013.* CDC, USDHHS. Available at: https://www.cdc.gov/aging/pdf/state-aging-health-in-america-2013.pdf Accessed December 3, 2022.

CDC. (2020). *CDC data show disproportionate COVID-19 impact in American Indian/Alaska Native populations*. Available at: https://www.cdc.gov/media/releases/2020/p0819-covid-19-impact-american-indian-alaska-native.html Accessed December 13, 2022.

CDC. (2021a). *Loneliness and social isolation linked to serious health conditions*. Available at: https://www.cdc.gov/aging/publications/features/lonely-older-adults.html. Accessed December 3, 2022.

CDC. (2021b). Underlying cause of death, 1999–2019. *National Vital Statistics System – Mortality Data (2019) via CDC WONDER*. Available at: https://wonder.cdc.gov/ Accessed December 3, 2022.

CDC. (2022a). *Social Determinants of Health at CDC*. Available at: https://www.cdc.gov/about/sdoh/index.html. Accessed February 9, 2023.

CDC. (2022b). *COVID data tracker*. Available at: https://covid.cdc.gov/covid-data-tracker/#datatracker-home. Accessed December 3, 2022.

CDC. (2022c). *Risk for COVID-19 infection, hospitalization, and death by race/ethnicity*. Available at: https://stacks.cdc.gov/view/cdc/121338 Accessed December 3, 2022.

CDC. (2022d). *Trends in demographic characteristics of people receiving COVID-19 vaccinations in the United States*. Available at: https://covid.cdc.gov/covid-data-tracker/#vaccination-demographics-trends Accessed December 13, 2022

Centers for Disease Control (CDC). (2009). *The power of prevention: Chronic disease… the public health challenge of the 21st century*. CDC, United States Department of Health and Human Services (USDHHS). Available at: https://stacks.cdc.gov/view/cdc/5509. Accessed December 3, 2022.

Cheng, Z., & Li, Y. (2022). Racial and ethnic and income disparities in COVID-19 vaccination among Medicare beneficiaries. *Journal of the American Geriatrics Society*, *70*(9), 2638–2645. https://doi.org/10.1111/jgs.17920

Chodosh, J., Thorpe, L. E., & Trinh-Shevrin, C. (2018). Changing faces of cognitive impairment in the U.S.: Detection strategies for underserved communities. *American Journal of Preventive Medicine*, *54*(6), 842–844. https://doi.org/10.1016/j.amepre.2018.02.016

Conejero, I., Olié, E., Courtet, P., & Calati, R. (2018). Suicide in older adults: Current perspectives. *Clinical Interventions in Aging*, *13*, 691–699. https://doi.org/10.2147/CIA.S130670

Đoàn, L. N., Takata, Y., Sakuma, K. K., & Irvin, V. L. (2019). Trends in Clinical Research Including Asian American, Native Hawaiian, and Pacific Islander Participants Funded by the US National Institutes of Health, 1992 to 2018. *JAMA Network Open*, *2*(7), e197432. https://doi.org/10.1001/jamanetworkopen.2019.7432

Dunlop, D. D., Song, J., Lyons, J. S., Manheim, L. M., & Chang, R. W. (2003). Racial/ethnic differences in rates of depression among preretirement adults. *American Journal of Public Health*, *93*(11), 1945–1952. https://doi.org/10.2105/ajph.93.11.1945

Feeding America. (2016). Executive summary: Spotlight on senior health adverse health outcomes of food insecurity in older Americans. *National Foundation to End Senior Hunger*. Available at: http://www.feedingamerica.org/hunger-in-america/our-research/senior-hunger-research/or-spotlight-on-senior-health-executive-summary.pdf. Accessed November 29, 2021.

Fitzgerald, N., Hromi-Fiedler, A., Segura-Pérez, S., & Pérez-Escamilla, R. (2011). Food insecurity is related to increased risk of type 2 diabetes among Latinas. *Ethnicity & Disease*, *21*(3), 328–334.

Forman, D. E., Maurer, M. S., Boyd, C., Brindis, R., Salive, M. E., Horne, F. M., Bell, S. P., Fulmer, T., Reuben, D. B., Zieman, S., & Rich, M. W. (2018). Multimorbidity in older adults with cardiovascular disease. *Journal of the American College of Cardiology*, *71*(19), 2149–2161. https://doi.org/10.1016/j.jacc.2018.03.022

Gawthrop, E. (2023) The color of Coronavirus: COVID-19 deaths by race and ethnicity in the U.S. *APM Research Lab*. Available at: https://www.apmresearchlab.org/covid/deaths-by-race. Accessed February 12, 2023

Gee, G. C., Ro, A., Shariff-Marco, S., & Chae, D. (2009). Racial discrimination and health among Asian Americans: Evidence, assessment, and directions for future research. *Epidemiologic Reviews*, *31*, 130–151. https://doi.org/10.1093/epirev/mxp009

Geronimus, A. T., Hicken, M., Keene, D., & Bound, J. (2006). "Weathering" and age patterns of allostatic load scores among blacks and whites in the United States. *American Journal of Public Health*, *96*(5), 826–833. https://doi.org/10.2105/AJPH.2004.060749

Goodman, R. A., Ling, S. M., Briss, P. A., Parrish, R. G., Salive, M. E., & Finke, B. S. (2016). Multimorbidity patterns in the United States: Implications for research and clinical practice. *The Journals of Gerontology. Series A, Biological Sciences and Medical Sciences*, *71*(2), 215–220. https://doi.org/10.1093/gerona/glv199

Gundersen, C., & Ziliak, J. P. (2015). Food insecurity and health outcomes. *Health Affairs*, *34*, 1830-1839. https://doi.org/10.1377/hlthaff.2015.0645

Hebert, L. E., Weuve, J., Scherr, P. A., & Evans, D. A. (2013). Alzheimer disease in the United States (2010–2050) estimated using the 2010 census. *Neurology*, *80*(19), 1778–1783. https://doi.org/10.1212/WNL.0b013e31828726f5

Hooker, K., Phibbs, S., Irvin, V. L., Mendez-Luck, C. A., Doan, L. N., Li, T., Turner, S., & Choun, S. (2019). Depression among older adults in the United States by disaggregated race and ethnicity. *The Gerontologist*, *59*(5), 886–891. https://doi.org/10.1093/geront/gny159

Joo, J. Y., & Liu, M. F. (2020). Culturally tailored interventions for ethnic minorities: A scoping review. *Nursing Open*, *8*(5), 2078–2090. https://doi.org/10.1002/nop2.733

Kalyanaraman Marcello, R., Dolle, J., Tariq, A., Kaur, S., Wong, L., Curcio, J., Thachil, R., Yi, S. S., & Islam, N. (2022). Disaggregating Asian race reveals COVID-19 disparities among Asian American Patients at New York City's public hospital system. *Public Health Reports (Washington, D.C. : 1974) 137*(2), 317–325. https://doi.org/10.1177/00333549211061313

Kenning, C., Daker-White, G., Blakemore, A., Panagioti, M., & Waheed, W. (2017). Barriers and facilitators in accessing dementia care by ethnic minority groups: A meta-synthesis of qualitative studies. *BMC Psychiatry*, *17*(1), 316. https://doi.org/10.1186/s12888-017-1474-0

Livingston, G., Sommerlad, A., Orgeta, V., Costafreda, S. G., Huntley, J., Ames, D., Ballard, C., Banerjee, S., Burns, A., Cohen-Mansfield, J., Cooper, C., Fox, N., Gitlin, L. N., Howard, R., Kales, H. C., Larson, E. B., Ritchie, K., Rockwood, K., Sampson, E. L., ... Mukadam, N. (2017). Dementia prevention, intervention, and care. *Lancet (London, England)*, *390*(10113), 2673–2734. https://doi.org/10.1016/S0140-6736(17)31363-6

Matthews, K. A., Xu, W., Gaglioti, A. H., Holt, J. B., Croft, J. B., Mack, D., & McGuire, L. C. (2019). Racial and ethnic estimates of Alzheimer's disease and related dementias in the United States (2015–2060) in adults aged ≥65 years. *Alzheimer's & Dementia: The Journal of the Alzheimer's Association*, *15*(1), 17–24. https://doi.org/10.1016/j.jalz.2018.06.3063

Mayeda, E. R., Glymour, M. M., Quesenberry, C. P., Jr, & Whitmer, R. A. (2017). Heterogeneity in 14-year Dementia Incidence Between Asian American Subgroups. *Alzheimer Disease and Associated Disorders*, *31*(3), 181–186. https://doi.org/10.1097/WAD.0000000000000189

McGrath, R. P., Snih, S. A., Markides, K. S., Faul, J. D., Vincent, B. M., Hall, O. T., & Peterson, M. D. (2019). The burden of health conditions across race and ethnicity for aging Americans: Disability-adjusted life years. *Medicine*, *98*(46), e17964. https://doi.org/10.1097/MD.0000000000017964

Medicare Payment Advisory Council. (2012 Mar). Report to congress medicare payment policy. *Hospice services*. 288. Available at: https://books.google.pt/books?hl=en&lr=&id=rr_O6ZOHo7sC&oi=fnd&pg=PR5&ots=7L2×7KdfJv&sig=YifhHlAI_pu0h9hs7XtBaOQX5Fw&redir_esc=y#v=onepage&q&f=false. Accessed December 3, 2022.

Menkin, J. A., Guan, S. A., Araiza, D., Reyes, C. E., Trejo, L., Choi, S. E., Willis, P., Kotick, J., Jimenez, E., Ma, S., McCreath, H. E., Chang, E., Witarama, T., & Sarkisian, C. A. (2017). Racial/Ethnic differences in expectations regarding aging among older adults. *The Gerontologist*, *57*(suppl_2), S138–S148. https://doi.org/10.1093/geront/gnx078

Moon, H., Badana, A., Hwang, S. Y., Sears, J. S., & Haley, W. E. (2019). Dementia Prevalence in Older Adults: Variation by Race/Ethnicity and Immigrant Status. *The American Journal of Geriatric Psychiatry: Official Journal of the American Association for Geriatric Psychiatry*, *27*(3), 241–250. https://doi.org/10.1016/j.jagp.2018.11.003

National Academies of Sciences. Engineering, and Medicine; Division of Behavioral and Social Sciences and Education; Health and Medicine Division; Board on Behavioral, Cognitive, and Sensory Sciences; Board on Health Sciences Policy; Committee on the Health and Medical Dimensions of Social Isolation and Loneliness in Older Adults. (2020). Social Isolation and Loneliness in Older Adults: Opportunities for the Health Care System. National Academies Press (US).

National Alliance for Caregiving & AARP Public Policy Institute. (2015). Caregiving in the U.S. Available at: https://www.aarp.org/content/dam/aarp/ppi/2015/caregiving-in-the-united-states-2015-report-revised.pdf. Accessed December 3, 2022.

National Institute on Aging (2019). National plan to address Alzheimer's disease: 2019 Update. Available at: https://aspe.hhs.gov/report/national-plan-address-alzheimers-disease-2019-update. Accessed December 3, 2022.

Ndugga, N., Hill, L., & Artiga, S. COVID-19 cases and deaths, vaccinations, and treatments by Race/Ethnicity as of Fall 2022. *Kaiser Family Foundation*. Available at: https://www.kff.org/racial-equity-and-health-policy/issue-brief/covid-19-cases-and-deaths-vaccinations-and-treatments-by-race-ethnicity-as-of-fall-2022 Accessed December 13, 2022

Niles, M. T., Beavers, A. W., Clay, L. A., Dougan, M. M., Pignotti, G. A., Rogus, S., Savoie-Roskos, M. R., Schattman, R. E., Zack, R. M., Acciai, F., Allegro, D., Belarmino, E. H., Bertmann, F., Biehl, E., Birk, N.,

Bishop-Royse, J., Bozlak, C., Bradley, B., Brenton, B. P., ... Yerxa, K. (2021). A Multi-Site Analysis of the Prevalence of Food Insecurity in the United States, before and during the COVID-19 Pandemic. *Current Developments in Nutrition, 5*(12), nzab135. https://doi.org/10.1093/cdn/nzab135.

Office of the Surgeon General, Center for Mental Health Services, & National Institute on Mental Health. (2001). Chapter 4 Mental Health for American Indians and Alaska Natives in Mental Health: Culture, Race, and Ethnicity. Substance Abuse and Mental Health Services Administration.

Quiñones, A. R., Botoseneanu, A., Markwardt, S., Nagel, C. L., Newsom, J. T., Dorr, D. A., & Allore, H. G. (2019). Racial/ethnic differences in multimorbidity development and chronic disease accumulation for middle-aged adults. *PloS One, 14*(6), e0218462. https://doi.org/10.1371/journal.pone.0218462

Rabbitt, M. P., Smith, M. D., & Coleman-Jensen, A. (2016). Food insecurity and hispanic diversity. Available at: https://www.ers.usda.gov/amber-waves/2016/july/food-insecurity-and-hispanic-diversity. Accessed December 3, 2022

Sadarangani, T. R., Missaelides, L., Yu, G., Trinh-Shevrin, C., & Brody, A. (2019a). Racial disparities in nutritional risk among community-dwelling older adults in adult day health care. *Journal of Nutrition in Gerontology and Geriatrics, 38*(4), 345–360. https://doi.org/10.1080/21551197.2019.1647327

Sadarangani, T. R., Salcedo, V., Chodosh, J., Kwon, S., Trinh-Shevrin, C., & Yi, S. (2020). Redefining the care continuum to create a pipeline to dementia care for minority populations. *Journal of Primary Care & Community Health, 11*, 2150132720921680. https://doi.org/10.1177/2150132720921680

Sadarangani, T. R., Trinh-Shevrin, C., Chyun, D., Yu, G., & Kovner, C. (2019b). Cardiovascular risk in middle-aged and older immigrants: Exploring residency period and health insurance coverage. *Journal of Nursing Scholarship: An Official Publication of Sigma Theta Tau International Honor Society of Nursing, 51*(3), 326–336. https://doi.org/10.1111/jnu.12465

Salive, M. E. (2013). Multimorbidity in older adults. *Epidemiologic Reviews, 35*, 75–83. https://doi.org/10.1093/epirev/mxs009

Spence, N. J., Adkins, D. E., & Dupre, M. E. (2011). Racial differences in depression trajectories among older women: Socioeconomic, family, and health influences. *Journal of Health and Social Behavior, 52*(4), 444–459.

Stanford, F. C. (2020). The importance of diversity and inclusion in the healthcare workforce. *Journal of the National Medical Association, 112*(3), 247–249. https://doi.org/10.1016/j.jnma.202.03.014.

Taylor, R. J., Chatters, L. M., & Taylor, H. O. (2019). Race and objective social isolation: Older African Americans, Black Caribbeans, and Non-Hispanic whites. *The Journals of Gerontology. Series B, Psychological Sciences and Social Sciences, 74*(8), 1429–1440. https://doi.org/10.1093/geronb/gby114

United States Census Bureau. (2020) Population estimates show aging across race groups differs. Available at: https://www.census.gov/newsroom/press-releases/2020/65-older-population-grows.html Accessed December 3, 2022.

United States Department of Health and Human Services. (2019). *National plan to address Alzheimer's disease: 2019 update.* Available at: https://aspe.hhs.gov/report/national-plan-address-alzheimers-disease-2019-update. Accessed December 3, 2022.

Williams, D. R., & Collins, C. (2001). Racial residential segregation: A fundamental cause of racial disparities in health. *Public Health Reports (Washington, D.C. : 1974) 116*(5), 404–416. https://doi.org/10.1093/phr/116.5.404

Wray, L. A., Alwin, D. F., & McCammon, R. J. (2005). Social status and risky health behaviors: Results from the health and retirement study. *The Journals of Gerontology. Series B, Psychological Sciences and Social Sciences, 60*(Spec No 2), 85–92. https://doi.org/10.1093/geronb/60.special_issue_2.s85

Yang, L. H., & WonPat-Borja, A. J. (2007). Psychopathology among Asian Americans. In F. T. L. Leong, et al. (Eds.), Handbook of Asian American psychology (pp. 379–405). Sage.

Zayas, C. E., He, Z., Yuan, J., Maldonado-Molina, M., Hogan, W., Modave, F., Guo, Y., & Bian, J. (2016). Examining healthcare utilization patterns of elderly middle-aged adults in the United States. *Proceedings of the ... International Florida AI Research Society Conference. Florida AI Research Symposium, 2016*, 361–366.

CHAPTER

UNDERSTANDING THE IMPACT OF THE SOCIAL DETERMINANTS OF HEALTH ON COGNITIVE HEALTH AMONG THE AGING POPULATION

JIAQI YANG, RACHEL SACKS, BEI WU, OMONIGHO MICHAEL BUBU, LU HU

LEARNING OBJECTIVES

By the end of this chapter, readers will be able to:

- Define the social determinants of health (SDOH).
- Describe ways in which an SDOH framework can guide research on aging and health.
- Describe early evidence related to the impact of SDOH on aging and cognitive health disparities.

Population Science Methods and Approaches to Aging and Alzheimer's Disease and Related Dementias Research, First Edition. Edited by Chau Trinh-Shevrin.
© 2024 John Wiley & Sons, Inc. Published 2024 by John Wiley & Sons, Inc.

INTRODUCTION

As described in the first chapter, Alzheimer's disease and Alzheimer's disease-related dementias (AD/ADRD) represent a growing global public health concern that disproportionately impacts people 65 years of age and older (Nichols et al., 2022; Wolters & Arfan Ikram, 2018). Research consistently demonstrates racial and ethnic disparities in AD/ADRD incidence and prevalence, with non-Hispanic Black (Black) and Hispanic (Latine) communities in particular demonstrating poorer cognitive health outcomes and disproportionately higher AD/ADRD prevalence than the non-Hispanic White (White) population (Alzheimer's Association, 2021). Because dementia is hypothesized to arise from a combination of biological, genetic, behavioral, and environmental factors over an individual's life course, there has been an increasing call for studies investigating the role of the social determinants of health (SDOH) in aging and dementia outcomes (Centers for Disease Control and Prevention, n.d.; Martin et al., 2021; Resende et al., 2019). Extant research suggests SDOH-related barriers contribute to disparities in cognitive health outcomes (Majoka & Schimming, 2021) but more research is needed to inform researchers and policymakers regarding what studies have already been undertaken and what gaps persist in the field. A better understanding of the ways in which SDOH impact AD/ADRD outcomes among older Americans could elucidate promising prevention, treatment, and supportive care strategies that are tailored to the socioeconomic, cultural, linguistic, and other attributes of the communities experiencing a disproportionate burden of AD/ADRD. This chapter will describe SDOH and serve as an introduction to this emerging realm of research. Chapter 3 will then build upon this introduction to discuss the impact of specific SDOH factors in greater detail through the lens of systemic racism and bias.

DEFINITIONS AND FRAMEWORK FOR UNDERSTANDING SDOH

SDOH are the environmental, social, economic, and psychosocial factors that affect people's health and health outcomes (Braveman & Gottlieb, 2014; Healthy People 2030, US Department of Health and Human Services, n.d.). The Healthy People initiative, which guides United States (US) federal policy related to disease prevention and health promotion and is revised every decade based on evolving health needs, defines SDOH as "the conditions in the environments where people are born, live, learn, work, play, worship, and age that affect a wide range of health functioning, and quality-of-life outcomes and risks" (Healthy People 2030, US Department of Health and Human Services, n.d.). SDOH are fundamental aspects of daily life that have profound impacts on individuals' well-being and are associated with the development and progression of many chronic diseases, including AD/ADRD, such as stable housing, adequate access to food and nutrition, safe neighborhoods, and affordable access to quality health care (Hill-Briggs et al., 2020; Majoka & Schimming, 2021; Powell-Wiley et al., 2022). The SDOH literature has grown rapidly over the last few decades (Berger & Gittlen, 2022; Davidson et al., 2021; Donkin et al., 2018), with both national and international organizations calling for increased screening and intervention related to SDOH-related factors as an essential way to promote health equity and improve health outcomes. The World Health Organization (WHO), the US National Institutes of Health (NIH), US Centers for Disease Control and Prevention (CDC), and US National Academies of Sciences, Engineering, and Medicine (NASEM) have established committees and workgroups to review evidence on SDOH and provide recommended actions (CDC, 2021; National Institute on Minority Health and Health Disparities, 2017; World Health Organization, 2010). In the United States, one of the five overarching goals of Healthy People 2030 is to "create social, physical, and economic environments that promote attaining the full potential for health and well-being for all" (Healthy People 2030, US Department of Health and Human Services, n.d.).

Toward this end, Healthy People 2030 identifies five domains that comprise a framework for studying these individual SDOH factors: 1) economic stability, 2) education access and quality, 3) health care access and quality, 4) neighborhood and built environment, and 5) social and community context (Figure 2.1).

The five domains, and factors within each domain, are interdependent and interconnected (Healthy People 2030, US Department of Health and Human Services, n.d.; Powell-Wiley et al., 2022). Examining these domains and factors holistically, identifying root causes, and designing interventions to address fundamental barriers will be essential to reducing disparities in health outcomes among diverse population groups (Braveman & Gottlieb, 2014). In the following sections, we will present each domain and introduce the ways in which these factors impact the health of older Americans.

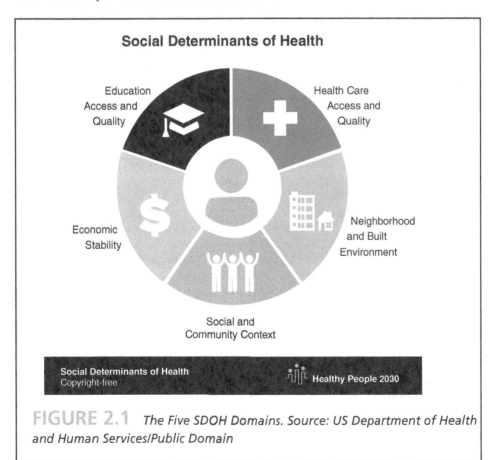

FIGURE 2.1   *The Five SDOH Domains. Source: US Department of Health and Human Services/Public Domain*

ECONOMIC STABILITY

The first domain, economic stability, significantly impacts all other domains and has pronounced system-level impacts on cognitive function and dementia risk (Braveman & Gottlieb, 2014; Powell-Wiley et al., 2022). It is strongly associated with other domains such as access to quality education and health care facilities, neighborhood environment, social networks, and support systems. Studies consistently suggest an association between lower economic status and a higher risk for AD/ADRD (Peterson et al., 2019; Samuel et al., 2020). For example, using data from the National Health and Aging Trends Study, researchers found that lower income was associated with a higher risk of incident dementia (Samuel et al., 2020). Lower economic status has also been linked to cognitive decline (Migeot et al., 2022; Peterson et al., 2019). In a large population-based study, Peterson and colleagues found that individuals with higher income had a much lower risk for cognitive decline than those with lower income (Peterson et al., 2019).

Race and ethnicity intersect with economic stability to impact health outcomes. Racial and ethnic minoritized groups continue to experience an enormous gap in income and wealth as compared to White people, with a significantly higher proportion of people who are members of racial and ethnic minoritized groups facing financial hardships. According to American Community Survey (ACS) five-year estimates, higher proportions of American Indian and Alaskan Native (AI/AN) (23.4%), Black (21.7%), Latine (17.7%), Native Hawaiian/Pacific Islander (16.7%), and Asian American (10.3%) families live below the poverty line as compared to White families (9.2%) (Ruggles et al., 2022). While the 2021 median household income was $75,412 for White people, the median was $72,234 for NH/PI people, $60,566 for Latine people, $46,221 for AI/AN people, and $46,679 for Black people (US Census Bureau, 2022a; Office of Minority Health 2022). Asian Americans had the highest median income, at $100,843, but this picture is complicated by substantial variation among subgroups, with some groups earning significantly less than others (US Census Bureau, 2022b). For example, while Indian American households had a mean income of $141,906, Burmese American households had a median income of $62,352. Moreover, 10 of the 16 Asian ethnic groups analyzed had poverty rates as high or higher than the average US household in 2021. It is also important to note that Asian American and NH/PI households typically are larger than White households, with multiple generations living under one roof, and tend to cluster in states with higher living expenses. NH/PI people also have a notably high average unemployment rate of 5.9% (Office of Minority Health, 2022). Immigration status also impacts income and economic stability, with pronounced effects on Latine, Asian American, and PI groups, in particular (Sudhinaraset et al., 2017).

Such differences in socioeconomic status may be important factors underpinning the racial disparities in cognitive health and AD/ADRD risk (Alzheimer's Association, 2021). For example, in a prospective study, Yaffe and colleagues found that Black people were more likely to develop dementia than White people; however, when the findings were adjusted for socioeconomic status, the racial difference for incident dementia was significantly reduced (Yaffe et al., 2013).

In addition to household income, occupation complexity and other aspects of employment have been considered as important predictors of AD/ADRD risks and outcomes (Hyun et al., 2022) and racially-based differences in occupation type, complexity, and job strain may influence AD/ADRD disparities. The associations between these employment-related factors and racially-based health disparities in cognitive decline and dementia outcomes are explored in greater detail in Chapter 3.

EDUCATION ACCESS AND QUALITY

Early childhood education, high school graduation, and college attendance are key factors in creating opportunities for individuals to achieve better paying jobs and greater economic stability and, consequently, safeguard other SDOH domains such as facilitating better access to quality health care. Children from low-income families, children with disabilities, and children who experience any form of discrimination are more likely to struggle in early education, setting them on a path toward lower educational attainment, less economic security, and greater risk of negative health outcomes, including chronic illnesses such as diabetes and depression (Office of Disease Prevention and Health Promotion, 2022a). Systemic racism is a key driver of disparities in education access and quality and is discussed in detail in Chapter 3.

Education has long been studied as a predictor of cognitive health function and AD/ADRD risk (Caamaño-Isorna et al., 2006; Zhang et al., 2009). Early studies suggested fewer years of education were associated with poorer cognitive function and higher risk of AD/ADRD (Caamaño-Isorna et al., 2006). One study found that fewer years of formal schooling predicted the risk of incident AD and that with each additional year of education, AD risk decreased by 17% (Evans et al., 1997). In a recent analysis of nationally representative data from the longitudinal Health and Retirement Study, the research team found that higher educational attainment was associated with higher cognition at baseline and that higher educational attainment significantly reduces the risk of cognitive decline (Clouston et al., 2020). It may be that education serves as a protective factor against neural damage. As posited by the cognitive reserve hypothesis (Stern, 2002, 2009), people have different capacities to cope with brain damage, arising from a combination of preexisting or compensatory cognitive processing approaches (Colombo et al., 2018) as well as different life experiences (Stern, 2002, 2009). A combination of these factors may impact dementia outcomes.

In line with this hypothesis, it is likely that racial and ethnic disparities in dementia outcomes derive, in part, from different and unequal life experiences and opportunities. Emerging evidence linking educational attainment and quality with racial and ethnic disparities in AD/ADRD outcomes is presented in Chapter 3.

HEALTH CARE ACCESS AND QUALITY

Access to timely, quality health care in the United States is associated inextricably with economic stability, educational attainment, and the neighborhood environment (Office of Disease Prevention and Health Promotion, 2022b). Abundant evidence links health insurance status, cost of care, and availability of primary and specialty care close to one's home with care-seeking and receipt of care (Baicker et al., 2013: Dickman et al., 2017; Franks et al., 1993). While research on associations between health care access and dementia outcomes is limited (Mukadam et al., 2013), emerging research suggests that limited access to quality health care may be linked to worse cognitive outcomes (Mullins et al., 2021). In their population-based study of aging Americans, Mullin and colleagues recently found that individuals living in an area with limited access to primary care and not having a regular source of care were associated with higher odds of cognitive impairment.

Racial and ethnic disparities in access to quality health care and services have been well documented (Caraballo et al., 2020; Fiscella & Sanders, 2016; Institute of Medicine 2003). Insurance status is a key factor in this equation. A 20-year analysis of National Health Interview Survey found that compared to White people, Black people and Latine people were more likely to be uninsured and experience cost-related barriers to care (Caraballo et al., 2020). Despite some narrowing of disparities among all racial and ethnic minoritized groups after the passage of the Affordable Care Act in 2010, Caraballo et al. found that rates of foregoing medical care because of cost have increased overall since 1999. Moreover, a ten-year analysis of American Community Survey data showed that uninsured rates were 7.8%, 7.4%, 11.4%, 20.0%, and 21.7% for nonelderly White, Asian American and NH/PI, Black, Latine, and AI/AN people, respectively (KFF, n.d -a). These differences were even more pronounced for employer-sponsored coverage. Compared to 65.8% of White and 64.8% of Asian American and NH/PI individuals having employer-based insurance coverage, only 47.2% of Black, 42.5% of Latine, and 36.6% of AI/AN individuals received insurance coverage from their employers (KFF, n.d.-b).

With respect to the impact of these trends on AD/ADRD outcomes, research has shown that Black and Latine people were more likely to receive a dementia diagnosis later in the disease trajectory and less likely to access dementia care, clinical trials, and medication (Co et al., 2021; Cooper et al., 2010; Luo et al., 2018). This is particularly disturbing given that the prevalence of AD/ADRD among Black and Latine people has been shown to be double and 1.5 times, respectively, that of White people (Alzheimer's Association, 2021; Quiñones et al., 2020). One recent analysis using data from 39 Alzheimer's Disease Research Centers (ADRCs) across the United States found that despite a documented higher risk of AD/ADRD among the Black population, Black patients were less likely to receive a dementia diagnosis than their White counterparts during their first medical visit to an ADRC (Suran, 2022). Another recent study used Consumer Assessment of Healthcare Providers and Systems (CAHPS) measures to assess patient-centeredness of care among patients from racial and ethnic minoritized group with AD/ADRD. Researchers found that patients belonging to any racial and ethnic minoritized group reported receiving worse quality of care and uncoordinated care, including lack of timely access to care, than White patients (Albaroudi & Chen, 2022). The role of structural racism and discrimination in limiting health care access for racialized and minoritized populations is further discussed in Chapter 3.

NEIGHBORHOOD AND BUILT ENVIRONMENT

Neighborhood and the built environment refers to a composite measure that captures level of neighborhood disadvantage as well as the physical environment of streets, sidewalks, buildings, parks, and other infrastructure in which people live (Besser et al., 2021; Powell et al., 2020). This measure is linked to other SDOH (e.g., economic stability, education access) and has been associated with chronic disease outcomes including cardiovascular disease and depression (Freedman et al., 2011; Yue et al., 2022), particularly in older people (Andrews et al., 2021; Nordstrom et al., 2004). Emerging research suggests links between the neighborhood and built environment and cognitive health outcomes, including AD/ADRD. Neighborhood deprivation, as measured by the Area Deprivation Index – a validated composite measure of 17 SDOH – has been associated with development of AD/ADRD (Hunt et al., 2020) as well as with increased risk for AD neuropathy (Powell et al., 2020).

Individual environmental factors included in this index have also been associated independently with cognitive health outcomes, including neighborhood walkability, food insecurity, and exposure to air pollutants. With regard to neighborhood walkability, one study of a multiethnic cohort found that individuals living in a neighborhood with numerous walking destinations were 1.24 times more likely to have improved cognition as compared to those with no walking destinations in their immediate area (Besser et al., 2021). Recent data show racial and ethnic disparities in walkability, with lower-income Black neighborhoods, particularly in the South, having lower walkability than majority White, Latine, Asian American and NH/PI neighborhoods (Conderino et al., 2021).

With respect to food insecurity, although researchers have not yet linked this factor directly to dementia, people who are food insecure appear to have a higher risk of cognitive impairment, a condition considered increasingly to be a transitional preclinical phase of dementia (Koyanagi et al., 2019). For example, a systematic review of 30 international studies suggested that people experiencing food insecurity were more likely to develop depression and have poorer cognition compared to individuals who were food secure and that food insecurity was strongly related to mild cognitive impairment (McMichael et al., 2022). A South African study found that people with moderate food insecurity were 2.82 times more likely to experience mild cognitive impairment than those who were food-secure (Koyanagi et al., 2019). These findings take on additional significance in light of data illustrating high rates of food insecurity among racial and ethnic minoritized populations, including NH/PI and some Asian American ethnic groups (Becerra et al., 2018; Long et al., 2020). Since the advent of the novel coronavirus disease 2019 (COVID-19) pandemic, rates of food insecurity among US households have skyrocketed from 10% to between 25% and 30%, with even higher rates among the most vulnerable population groups, including older adults from racial and ethnic minoritized communities and those with limited English proficiency, including Black, Latine, and AI/AN populations (Niles et al., 2021; Otten et al., 2022; Tai-Seale et al., 2022).

Finally, with regard to air pollution, research suggests that chronic exposure to heavy metals emitted by such sources as gasoline, wildfires, contaminated soil, and waste processing facilities and carried by fine particulate matter ($PM_{2.5}$) is associated with negative cognitive health outcomes, including incident dementia and AD risk (Calderón-Garcidueñas et al., 2022). Long-term exposure to aluminum, copper, mercury, and lead in the air causes neurological disorders and damages nerve fibers and glial cells – changes that may increase the risk of dementia (Antoniadou et al., 2020). More research is needed to better understand these links.

Racial residential segregation is associated with health disparities, including racial disparities in cognitive health outcomes (Pohl et al., 2021). Yet segregation may serve both as a mediator and moderator of dementia risk and incidence. Although racially segregated areas with residents from predominantly minoritized groups typically face higher resource deprivation, these communities may also demonstrate greater social cohesion, which can positively impact cognitive health outcomes (Pohl et al., 2021). For non-Black minoritized communities, researchers have suggested there may be a protective effect of residing in an ethnic enclave, particularly for recent immigrants, people with low English proficiency (LEP), and AI/AN people living near or on reservations (González Burchard et al., 2005; Wong et al., 2020). The data, however, remain inconclusive (González Burchard et al., 2005; Kim et al., 2014).

Chapter 3 discusses the impact of racism on historical residential segregation and reviews this evidence in greater detail.

SOCIAL AND COMMUNITY CONTEXT

Level of social engagement, measured by number of social contacts and social networks, is another critical factor in SDOH. Aspects of social engagement include relationships and interactions with family, friends, co-workers, and community members – connections that can have positive or negative impacts on an individual's health and well-being (Office of Disease Prevention and Health Promotion, 2022c). Whereas many people receive the social support they need from these relationships and interactions, other people lack these connections or face challenging situations at home, work, or school. Interventions that help build social and community networks for these individuals can be helpful in reinforcing health-promoting behaviors and outcomes. Examples of such interventions include art and dance classes for older adults in senior centers, after-school activities for at-risk children and youth, mobile/online network-building, voter registration outreach, and employment counseling programs.

Research suggests that strong social and community connections may be protective against age-related cognitive decline, irrespective of race and ethnicity (Barnes et al., 2004; Lamar et al., 2022; Samuel et al., 2015). For example, one cohort study with a majority of Black participants showed that a higher frequency of social networking with families and friends or participating in social activities was linked to a decreased rate of cognitive decline in older age for all participants (Barnes et al., 2004). Similarly, but conversely, a longitudinal study of Japanese Americans showed that weak social networks were associated with increased incidence of all-cause dementia as well as AD, but not vascular dementia (Kallianpur et al., 2022). The importance of social and community ties may persist even among the oldest members of a given population. A Swedish cohort study concluded that for individuals older than 85 years, those with more social contacts were 17% less likely to develop dementia after five years of follow-up (Wallin et al., 2013). These findings are in line with the cognitive reserve hypothesis that mental stimulation during midlife render the brain more resistant to cognitive decline later in life. More research is needed to explore this hypothesis.

Additionally, more research is needed to better understand the reciprocal relationship between AD/ADRD and social networks. While stronger social networks may be protective against cognitive decline, dementia contributes to social loss among older people – a process that, in turn, worsens cognitive decline (Sachdev, 2022). Thus, although implementing programs and mechanisms to strengthen social networks among people in middle and later life may be effective as components in a constellation of strategies to prevent the onset of AD/ADRD, preserving these networks or building new social connections may be less useful as care strategies to support older people already diagnosed with AD/ADRD.

SUMMARY

Given that AD/ADRD is hypothesized to result from a combination of biological, genetic, behavioral, and environmental factors experienced throughout the life course, there is an urgent need for more research to elucidate the complex role that SDOH play in impacting aging and dementia outcomes. Existing data have suggested links between modifiable SDOH (e.g., $PM_{2.5}$ level) and cognitive health outcomes (e.g., incident dementia). Community-engaged study designs may be particularly helpful in this regard because participatory methodologies allow researchers to work hand-in-hand with diverse communities to develop, implement, and evaluate findings that can then inform program and policy responses. Indeed, an important aspect of the next phase of SDOH and cognitive health research should be to explore the effects of various factors within a single socioeconomic stratum, racial or ethnic group, or geographic area in order to elucidate intragroup associations. As the aging population diversifies, these types of studies will prove essential to understanding cognitive health in distinct population groups experiencing health disparities, such as racial and ethnic minoritized groups, LEP populations, and rural communities. Finally, it is notable that at present, systems-level intervention studies aiming to improve SDOH are scarce, with most interventions focusing on individual-level behavior change. Establishing multisectoral collaborations to address structural racism, historical socioeconomic deprivation, and other upstream factors impacting SDOH will be essential to reducing health disparities, including dementia outcomes, as well as ensuring equity and promoting better health among racial and ethnically diverse older populations.

DISCUSSION QUESTIONS

1. What are SDOH?

2. Why it is important to consider SDOH when evaluating the health of the aging population?

3. What are some individual SDOH factors that may contribute to disparities in cognitive health and dementia among diverse population groups in the United States?

REFERENCES

Albaroudi, A., & Chen, J. (2022). Consumer assessment of healthcare providers and systems among racial and ethnic minority patients with Alzheimer disease and related dementias. *JAMA Network Open, 5*(9),e2233436. PMID: 36166229; PMCID: PMC9516284. https://doi.org/10.1001/jamanetworkopen.2022.33436

Alzheimer's Association. (2021). 2021 Alzheimer's disease facts and figures. *Alzheimer's & Dementia: The Journal of the Alzheimer's Association, 17*(3), 327–406. https://doi.org/10.1002/alz.12328

Andrews, M. R., Ceasar, J., Tamura, K., Langerman, S. D., Mitchell, V. M., Collins, B. S., Baumer, Y., Gutierrez Huerta, C. A., Dey, A. K., Playford, M. P., Mehta, N. N., & Powell-Wiley, T. M. (2021). Neighborhood environment perceptions associate with depression levels and cardiovascular risk among middle-aged and older adults: Data from the Washington, DC cardiovascular health and needs assessment. *Aging & Mental Health, 25*(11), 2078–2089. https://doi.org/10.1080/13607863.2020.1793898

Antoniadou, F., Papamitsou, T., Kavvadas, D., Kapoukranidou, D., Sioga, A., & Papaliagkas, V. (2020). Toxic environmental factors and their association with the development of dementia: A mini review on heavy metals and ambient particulate matter. *Materia Socio-Medica, 32*(4), 299. https://doi.org/10.5455/msm.2020.32.299-306

Austin, A. (2022). A brief look at low-income Asian Americans and pacific Islanders. Available at: https://cepr.net/a-brief-look-at-low-income-asian-americans-and-pacific-islanders Accessed December 8, 2022

Baicker, K., Taubman, S. L., Allen, H. L., Bernstein, M., Gruber, J. H., Newhouse, J. P., ... Finkelstein, A. N. (2013). The Oregon experiment — Effects of Medicaid on clinical outcomes. *New England Journal of Medicine, 368*(18), 1713–1722. https://doi.org/10.1056/NEJMsa1212321

Barnes, L. L., Mendes de Leon, C., Wilson, R., Bienias, J., & Evans, D. (2004). Social resources and cognitive decline in a population of older African Americans and whites. *Neurology, 63*(12), 2322–2326. https://doi.org/10.1212/01.wnl.0000147473.04043.b3

Becerra, M. B., Mshigeni, S. K., & Becerra, B. J. (2018). The Overlooked Burden of Food Insecurity among Asian Americans: Results from the California health interview survey. *International Journal of Environmental Research and Public Health, 15*(8), 1684. https://doi.org/10.3390/ijerph15081684

Berger, D. H., & Gittlen, S. (2022). Addressing social determinants of health requires stronger public-private alliances. *NEJM Catalyst Innovations in Care Delivery, 3*(1). https://doi.org/10.1056/CAT.21.0435

Besser, L. M., Chang, L. C., Hirsch, J. A., Rodriguez, D. A., Renne, J., Rapp, S. R., ... Hughes, T. M. (2021). Longitudinal associations between the neighborhood built environment and cognition in US older adults: The multi-ethnic study of atherosclerosis. *International Journal of Environmental Research Public Health, 18*(15). https://doi.org/10.3390/ijerph18157973

Braveman, P., & Gottlieb, L. (2014). The social determinants of health: It's time to consider the causes of the causes. *Public Health Reports, 129*(Suppl 2), 19. https://doi.org/10.1177/00333549141291S206

Bryant, R. T.-A.-F. (2015). *College Preparation for African American Students: Gaps in the High School Educational Experience.* Retrieved from https://cdn.uncf.org/wp-content/uploads/PDFs/College-readiness2-2.pdf?_ga=2.191016685.618341616.1664472907-867261817.1664472907

Caamaño-Isorna, F., Corral, M., Montes-Martínez, A., & Takkouche, B. (2006). Education and dementia: A meta-analytic study. *Neuroepidemiology, 26*(4), 226–232. https://doi.org/10.1159/000093378

Calderón-Garcidueñas, L., Chávez-Franco, D. A., Luévano-Castro, S. C., Macías-Escobedo, E., Hernández-Castillo, A., Carlos-Hernández, E., Franco-Ortíz, A., Castro-Romero, S. P., Cortés-Flores, M., Crespo-Cortés, C. N., Torres-Jardón, R., Stommel, E. W., Rajkumar, R. P., & Mukherjee, P. S., & Research Universidad del Valle de México UVM Group. (2022). Metals, nanoparticles, particulate matter, and cognitive decline. *Frontiers in Neurology, 12*, 794071. https://doi.org/10.3389/fneur.2021.794071

Caraballo, C., Massey, D., Mahajan, S., Lu, Y., Annapureddy, A. R., Roy, B., … Krumholz, H. M. (2020). Racial and ethnic disparities in access to health care among adults in the United States: A 20-Year national health interview survey analysis, 1999-2018. *MedRxiv : The Preprint Server for Health Sciences.* https://doi.org/10.1101/2020.10.30.20223420

CDC. (2021). *Social Determinants of Health | CDC.* Retrieved September 21, 2021, from https://www.cdc.gov/socialdeterminants/index.htm

Centers for Disease Control and Prevention. (n.d.). Social determinants of health and Alzheimer's disease and related dementias. Retrieved October 13, 2022, from https://www.cdc.gov/aging/disparities/social-determinants-alzheimers.html

Clouston, S. A. P., Smith, D. M., Mukherjee, S., Zhang, Y., Hou, W., Link, B. G., & Richards, M. (2020). Education and cognitive decline: An integrative analysis of global longitudinal studies of cognitive aging. *The Journals of Gerontology Series B: Psychological Sciences and Social Sciences, 75*(7), e151. https://doi.org/10.1093/GERONB/GBZ053

Co, M., Couch, E., Gao, Q., Mac-Ginty, S., Das-Munshi, J., & Prina, M. (2021). Access to health services in older minority ethnic groups with dementia: A systematic review. *Journal of the American Geriatrics Society, 69*(3), 822–834. https://doi.org/10.1111/JGS.16929

Colombo, B., Antonietti, A., & Daneau, B. (2018). The relationships between cognitive reserve and creativity. A study on American aging population. *Frontiers in Psychology, 9*. https://doi.org/10.3389/fpsyg.2018.00764

Conderino, S. E., Feldman, J. M., Spoer, B., Gourevitch, M. N., & Thorpe, L. E. (2021). Social and economic differences in neighborhood walkability across 500 U.S. cities. *American Journal of Preventive Medicine, 61*(3), 394–401. https://doi.org/10.1016/j.amepre.2021.03.014

Cooper, C., Tandy, A. R., Balamurali, T. B. S., & Livingston, G. (2010). A systematic review and meta-analysis of ethnic differences in use of dementia treatment, care, and research. *The American Journal of Geriatric Psychiatry : Official Journal of the American Association for Geriatric Psychiatry, 18*(3), 193–203. https://doi.org/10.1097/JGP.0B013E3181BF9CAF

Davidson, K. W., Krist, A. H., Tseng, C.-W., Simon, M., Doubeni, C. A., Kemper, A. R., … Borsky, A. (2021). Incorporation of social risk in US preventive services task force recommendations and identification of key challenges for primary care. *JAMA.* https://doi.org/10.1001/JAMA.2021.12833

Dickman, S. L., Himmelstein, D. U., & Woolhandler, S. (2017). Inequality and the health-care system in the USA. *Lancet (London, England), 389*(10077), 1431–1441. https://doi.org/10.1016/S0140-6736(17)30398-7

Donkin, A., Goldblatt, P., Allen, J., Nathanson, V., & Marmot, M. (2018). Global action on the social determinants of health. *BMJ global health, 3*(Suppl 1), e000603. https://doi.org/10.1136/bmjgh-2017-000603

Evans, D. A., Hebert, L. E., Beckett, L. A., Scherr, P. A., Albert, M. S., Chown, M. J., … Taylor, J. O. (1997). Education and other measures of socioeconomic status and risk of incident Alzheimer disease in a defined population of older persons. *Archives of Neurology, 54*(11), 1399–1405. https://doi.org/10.1001/ARCHNEUR.1997.00550230066019

Fiscella, K., & Sanders, M. R. (2016). Racial and ethnic disparities in the quality of health care. *Annual Review of Public Health, 37*, 375–394. https://doi.org/10.1146/annurev-publhealth-032315-021439

Franks, P., Clancy, C. M., & Gold, M. R. (1993). Health insurance and mortality: Evidence from a national cohort. *JAMA, 270*(6), 737–741. https://doi.org/10.1001/jama.1993.03510060083037

Freedman, V. A., Grafova, I. B., & Rogowski, J. (2011). Neighborhoods and chronic disease onset in later life. *American Journal of Public Health, 101*(1), 79–86. https://doi.org/10.2105/AJPH.2009.178640

González Burchard, E., Borrell, L. N., Choudhry, S., Naqvi, M., Tsai, H. J., Rodriguez-Santana, J. R., Chapela, R., Rogers, S. D., Mei, R., Rodriguez-Cintron, W., Arena, J. F., Kittles, R., Perez-Stable, E. J., Ziv, E., &

Risch, N. (2005). Latino Populations: A Unique Opportunity for the Study of Race, Genetics, and Social Environment in Epidemiological Research. *American Journal of Public Health*, *95*(12), 2161–2168. https://doi.org/10.2105/AJPH.2005.068668

Healthy People 2030, U.S. Department of Health and Human Services, O. of D. P. and H. P. (n.d.). Social determinants of health. Retrieved July 1, 2022, from https://health.gov/healthypeople/priority-areas/social-determinants-health

Hill-Briggs, F., Adler, N. E., Berkowitz, S. A., Chin, M. H., Gary-Webb, T. L., Navas-Acien, A., ... Haire-Joshu, D. (2020). Social determinants of health and diabetes: A scientific review. *Diabetes Care*, *44*(1), 258–279. https://doi.org/10.2337/dci20-0053

Hunt, J. F. V., Vogt, N. M., Jonaitis, E. M., Buckingham, W. R., Koscik, R. L., Zuelsdorff, M., ... Asthana, S. (2020). Neighborhood disadvantage is associated with accelerated cortical thinning and cognitive decline in cognitively unimpaired adults: Public health: ADRD risk and protective factors: Brain changes and mechanisms. *Alzheimer's & Dementia*, *16*(S10), e043170. https://doi.org/10.1002/alz.043170

Hyun, J., Hall, C. B., Katz, M. J., Derby, C. A., Lipnicki, D. M., Crawford, J. D., ... Lipton, R. B. (2022). Education, occupational complexity, and incident dementia: A COSMIC collaborative cohort study. *Journal of Alzheimer's Disease : JAD*, *85*(1), 179. https://doi.org/10.3233/JAD-210627

Institute of Medicine (U.S.) Committee on Understanding and Eliminating Racial and Ethnic Disparities in Health Care. (2003). *Unequal treatment: Confronting racial and ethnic disparities in health care* (B. D. Smedley, A. Y. Stith, & A. R. Nelson Eds.). National Academies Press.

Kallianpur, K. J., Masaki, K. H., Chen, R., Willcox, B. J., Allsopp, R. C., Davy, P., & Dodge, H. H. (2022). Weak social networks in late life predict incident Alzheimer's disease: The Kuakini Honolulu-Asia aging study. *The Journals of Gerontology. Series A, Biological Sciences and Medical Sciences*, glac215. Advance online publication. https://doi.org/10.1093/gerona/glac215

KFF. (n.d.-a). Uninsured rates for the Nonelderly by Race/Ethnicity | *KFF*. Retrieved October 13, 2022, from https://www.kff.org/uninsured/state-indicator/nonelderly-uninsured-rate-by-raceethnicity/?currentTimeframe=0&sortModel=%7B%22colId%22:%22Location%22,%22sort%22:%22asc%22%7D

KFF. (n.d.-b). *Employer-sponsored coverage rates for the nonelderly by Race/Ethnicity | KFF*. Retrieved October 13 2022, from https://www.kff.org/other/state-indicator/nonelderly-employer-coverage-rate-by-raceethnicity/?currentTimeframe=0&sortModel=%7B%22colId%22:%22Location%22,%22sort%22:%22asc%22%7D

Kim, Y. A., Collins, T. W., & Grineski, S. E. (2014). Neighborhood context and the Hispanic health paradox: Differential effects of immigrant density on children's wheezing by poverty, nativity and medical history. *Health & Place*, *27*, 1–8. https://doi.org/10.1016/j.healthplace.2014.01.006

Koyanagi, A., Veronese, N., Stubbs, B., Vancampfort, D., Stickley, A., Oh, H., ... Lara, E. (2019). Food insecurity is associated with mild cognitive impairment among middle-aged and older adults in South Africa: Findings from a nationally representative survey. *Nutrients*, *11*(4), 749. https://doi.org/10.3390/nu11040749

Lamar, M., James, B. D., Glover, C. M., Capuano, A. W., McSorley, V. E., Wilson, R. S., & Barnes, L. L. (2022). Social engagement and all-cause mortality: A focus on participants of the minority aging research study. *American Journal of Preventive Medicine*, *63*(5), 700–707. https://doi.org/10.1016/j.amepre.2022.05.005

Long, C. R., Rowland, B., McElfish, P. A., Ayers, B. L., & Narcisse, M. R. (2020). Food security status of native Hawaiians and Pacific Islanders in the US: Analysis of a national survey. *Journal of Nutrition Education and Behavior*, *52*(8), 788–795. https://doi.org/10.1016/j.jneb.2020.01.009

Luo, H. B., Yu, G., & Wu, B. (2018). Self-reported cognitive impairment across racial/ethnic groups in the United States, National health interview survey, 1997–2015. *Preventing Chronic Disease*. https://doi.org/10.5888/pcd15.170338

Majoka, M. A., & Schimming, C. (2021). Effect of social determinants of health on cognition and risk of Alzheimer disease and related Dementias. *Clinical Therapeutics*, *43*(6), 922–929. https://doi.org/10.1016/J.CLINTHERA.2021.05.005

Martin, R., Shan, L., Geldmacher, D., Pilonieta, G., Kennedy, R., Oates, G., ... Kinney, J. (2021). Social determinants of Alzheimer's disease and related Dementias: Racial and regional variations. *Innovation in Aging*, *5*(Supplement_1), 101–101. https://doi.org/10.1093/GERONI/IGAB046.382

McMichael, A. J., McGuinness, B., Lee, J., Minh, H. V., Woodside, J. V., & McEvoy, C. T. (2022). Food insecurity and brain health in adults: A systematic review. *Critical reviews in food science and nutrition*, *62*(31), 8728–8743. https://doi.org/10.1080/10408398.2021.1932721

Migeot, J., Calivar, M., Granchetti, H., Ibáñez, A., & Fittipaldi, S. (2022). Socioeconomic status impacts cognitive and socioemotional processes in healthy ageing. *Scientific Reports*, *12*(1), 1–11. https://doi.org/10.1038/s41598-022-09580-4

Mukadam, N., Cooper, C., & Livingston, G. (2013). Improving access to dementia services for people from minority ethnic groups. *Current Opinion in Psychiatry*, *26*(4), 409–414. https://doi.org/10.1097/YCO.0B013E32835EE668

Mullins, M. A., Bynum, J. P. W., Judd, S. E., & Clarke, P. J. (2021). Access to primary care and cognitive impairment: Results from a national community study of aging Americans. *BMC Geriatrics*, *21*(1), 1–10. https://doi.org/10.1186/S12877-021-02545-8/FIGURES/3

National Institute on Minority Health and Health Disparities. (2017). *NIMHD research framework*. Retrieved September 20, 2021, from https://www.nimhd.nih.gov/about/overview/research-framework/nimhd-framework.html

Nichols, E., Steinmetz, J. D., Vollset, S. E., Fukutaki, K., Chalek, J., Abd-Allah, F., ... Vos, T. (2022). Estimation of the global prevalence of dementia in 2019 and forecasted prevalence in 2050: An analysis for the global Burden of disease study 2019. *The Lancet Public Health*, *7*(2), e105–e125. https://doi.org/10.1016/S2468-2667(21)00249-8/ATTACHMENT/60E03FD1-38B2-4B40-A91D-9AFDDA22B45E/MMC1.PDF

Niles, M. T., Beavers, A. W., Clay, L. A., Dougan, M. M., Pignotti, G. A., Rogus, S., Savoie-Roskos, M. R., Schattman, R. E., Zack, R. M., Acciai, F., Allegro, D., Belarmino, E. H., Bertmann, F., Biehl, E., Birk, N., Bishop-Royse, J., Bozlak, C., Bradley, B., Brenton, B. P., ... Yerxa, K. (2021). A multi-site analysis of the prevalence of food insecurity in the United States, before and during the COVID-19 Pandemic. *Current Developments in Nutrition*, *5*(12), nzab135. https://doi.org/10.1093/cdn/nzab135

Nordstrom, C. K., Diez Roux, A. V., Jackson, S. A., & Gardin, J. M., & Cardiovascular Health Study. (2004). The association of personal and neighborhood socioeconomic indicators with subclinical cardiovascular disease in an elderly cohort. The cardiovascular health study. *Social Science & Medicine (1982)*, *59*(10), 2139–2147. https://doi.org/10.1016/j.socscimed.2004.03.017

Office of Disease Prevention and Health Promotion, Office of the Assistant Secretary for Health, Office of the Secretary, U.S. Department of Health and Human Services. (2022a). Education access and quality. Available at: https://health.gov/healthypeople/objectives-and-data/browse-objectives/education-access-and-quality. Accessed December 4, 2022

Office of Disease Prevention and Health Promotion, Office of the Assistant Secretary for Health, Office of the Secretary, U.S. Department of Health and Human Services. (2022b). Health care access and quality. Available at: https://health.gov/healthypeople/objectives-and-data/browse-objectives/health-care-access-and-quality. Accessed December 4, 2022

Office of Disease Prevention and Health Promotion, Office of the Assistant Secretary for Health, Office of the Secretary, U.S. Department of Health and Human Services. (2022c). *Social and community context*. Available at: https://health.gov/healthypeople/objectives-and-data/browse-objectives/social-and-community-context Accessed December 4, 2022

Office of Minority Health, U.S. Department of Health and Human Services. (2022). Profile: Native Hawaiians/Pacific Islanders. Available at: https://minorityhealth.hhs.gov/omh/browse.aspx?lvl=3&lvlid=65 Accessed December 8, 2022

Otten, J. J., Averill, M. M., & Spiker, M. L. (2022). Food security and food access during the COVID-19 pandemic: Impacts, adaptations, and looking ahead. *JPEN. Journal of Parenteral and Enteral Nutrition*, Advance online publication. 10.1002/jpen.2445. https://doi.org/10.1002/jpen.2445

Peterson, R. L., Carvajal, S. C., McGuire, L. C., Fain, M. J., & Bell, M. L. (2019). State inequality, socioeconomic position and subjective cognitive decline in the United States. *SSM - Population Health*, *7*, 100357. https://doi.org/10.1016/J.SSMPH.2019.100357

Pohl, D. J., Seblova, D., Avila, J. F., Dorsman, K. A., Kulick, E. R., Casey, J. A., & Manly, J. (2021). Relationship between residential segregation, later-life cognition, and incident dementia across race/ethnicity. *International Journal of Environmental Research and Public Health*, *18*(21), 11233. https://doi.org/10.3390/ijerph182111233

Powell, W. R., Buckingham, W. R., Larson, J. L., Vilen, L., Yu, M., Salamat, M. S., ... Kind, A. J. H. (2020). Association of neighborhood-level disadvantage with Alzheimer disease neuropathology. *JAMA Network Open*, *3*(6), e207559–e207559. https://doi.org/10.1001/jamanetworkopen.2020.7559

Powell-Wiley, T. M., Baumer, Y., Baah, F. O., Baez, A. S., Farmer, N., Mahlobo, C. T., ... Wallen, G. R. (2022). Social determinants of cardiovascular disease. *Circulation Research*, *130*(5), 782–799. https://doi.org/10.1161/CIRCRESAHA.121.319811

Quiñones, A. R., Kaye, J., Allore, H. G., Botoseneanu, A., & Thielke, S. M. (2020 Jan-Dec). An agenda for addressing multimorbidity and racial and ethnic disparities in Alzheimer's disease and related Dementia. *American Journal of Alzheimer's Disease Other Demen*, *35*, 1533317520960874. https://doi.org/10.1177/1533317520960874. PMID: 32969234; PMCID: PMC7984095.

Resende, E. D. P. F., Llibre Guerra, J. J., & Miller, B. L. (2019). Health and socioeconomic inequities as contributors to brain health. *JAMA Neurology*, *76*(6), 633–634. https://doi.org/10.1001/JAMANEUROL.2019.0362

Ruggles, S., Flood, S., Goeken, R., Schouweiler, M., & Sobek, M. (2022). IPUMS USA: Version 12.0 [2017–2021] American community survey 5-year estimates. IPUMS. https://doi.org/10.18128/D010.V12.0

Sachdev, P. S. (2022). Social health, social reserve and dementia. *Current Opinion in Psychiatry*, *35*(2), 111–117. https://doi.org/10.1097/YCO.0000000000000779

Samuel, L. J., Dennison Himmelfarb, C. R., Szklo, M., Seeman, T. E., Echeverria, S. E., & Diez Roux, A. V. (2015). Social engagement and chronic disease risk behaviors: The Multi-Ethnic Study of Atherosclerosis. *Preventive Medicine*, *71*, 61–66. https://doi.org/10.1016/j.ypmed.2014.12.008

Samuel, L. J., Szanton, S. L., Wolff, J. L., Ornstein, K. A., Parker, L. J., & Gitlin, L. N. (2020). Socioeconomic disparities in six-year incident dementia in a nationally representative cohort of U.S. older adults: An examination of financial resources. *BMC Geriatrics*, *20*(1), 1–9. https://doi.org/10.1186/S12877-020-01553-4/FIGURES/2

Stern, Y. (2002). What is cognitive reserve? Theory and research application of the reserve concept. *Journal of the International Neuropsychological Society*, *8*(3), 448–460. https://doi.org/10.1017/S1355617702813248

Stern, Y. (2009). Cognitive reserve. *Neuropsychologia*, *47*(10), 2015–2028. https://doi.org/10.1016/j.neuropsychologia.2009.03.004

Sudhinaraset, M., To, T. M., Ling, I., Melo, J., & Chavarin, J. (2017). The influence of deferred action for childhood arrivals on undocumented Asian and Pacific Islander young adults: Through a social determinants of health lens. *The Journal of Adolescent Health: Official Publication of the Society for Adolescent Medicine*, *60*(6), 741–746. https://doi.org/10.1016/j.jadohealth.2017.01.008

Suran, M. (2022). Racial disparities in dementia diagnoses. *JAMA*, *327*(8), 709–709. https://doi.org/10.1001/JAMA.2022.0979

Tai-Seale, M., Cheung, M. W., Kwak, J., Harris, V., Madonis, S., Russell, L., Haley, E., & Agnihotri, P. (2022). Unmet needs for food, medicine, and mental health services among vulnerable older adults during the COVID-19 pandemic. *Health Services Research*, Advance online publication, 10.1111/1475–6773.14084. https://doi.org/10.1111/1475-6773.14084

US Census Bureau. (2022a). *2021* American community survey 1-year estimates. Retrieved February 25, 2023, from https:https://www.census.gov/programs-surveys/acs/technical-documentation/table-and-geography-changes/2021/1-year.html

US Census Bureau. (2022b). Poverty in the United States: 2021. Retrieved October 13 2022, from https://www.census.gov/library/publications/2022/demo/p60-277.html

Wallin, K., Boström, G., Kivipelto, M., & Gustafson, Y. (2013). Risk factors for incident dementia in the very old. *International Psychogeriatrics*, *25*(7), 1135–1143. https://doi.org/10.1017/s1041610213000409

Wolters, F. J., & Arfan Ikram, M. (2018). Epidemiology of Dementia: The Burden on society, the challenges for research. *Methods in Molecular Biology (Clifton, N.J.)*, *1750*, 3–14. https://doi.org/10.1007/978-1-4939-7704-8_1

Wong, M. S., Steers, W. N., Hoggatt, K. J., Ziaeian, B., & Washington, D. L. (2020). Relationship of neighborhood social determinants of health on racial/ethnic mortality disparities in US veterans-Mediation and moderating effects. *Health Services Research*, *55*(Suppl 2), 851–862. https://doi.org/10.1111/1475-6773.13547

World Health Organization. (2010). A conceptual framework for action on the social determinants of health. Retrieved July 1, 2022, from https://www.who.int/publications/i/item/9789241500852

Yaffe, K., Falvey, C., Harris, T. B., Newman, A., Satterfield, S., Koster, A., … Simonsick, E. (2013). Effect of socioeconomic disparities on incidence of dementia among biracial older adults: Prospective study. *BMJ*, *347*. https://doi.org/10.1136/BMJ.F7051

Yue, X., Antonietti, A., Alirezaei, M., Tasdizen, T., Li, D., Nguyen, L., Mane, H., Sun, A., Hu, M., Whitaker, R. T., & Nguyen, Q. C. (2022). Using convolutional neural networks to derive neighborhood built environments from google street view images and examine their associations with health outcomes. *International Journal of Environmental Research and Public Health*, *19*(19), 12095. https://doi.org/10.3390/ijerph191912095

Zhang, Z. X., Plassman, B. L., Xu, Q., Zahner, G., Wu, B., Gai, M. Y., Wen, H. B., Chen, X., Gao, S., Hu, D., Xiao, X. H., Shen, Y., Liu, A. M., & Xu, T. (2009). Lifespan influences on mid-to late-life cognitive function in a Chinese birth cohort. *Neurology*, *73*(3), 186–194. PMCID: PMC2843580. https://doi.org/10.1212/WNL.0b013e3181ae7c90

CHAPTER

SYSTEMIC RACISM, DISCRIMINATION, AND STIGMA

RUIJIA CHEN, SUPRIYA MISRA

LEARNING OBJECTIVES

By the end of this chapter, readers will be able to:

- Identify key domains of structural racism and their specific impacts on disparities in cognitive aging and dementia.
- Consider how structural racism manifests in clinical and research processes through structural bias in assessment and diagnosis and exclusion from research.
- Describe the role of racial discrimination and stigma in cognitive aging and dementia.

Population Science Methods and Approaches to Aging and Alzheimer's Disease and Related Dementias Research, First Edition. Edited by Chau Trinh-Shevrin.
© 2024 John Wiley & Sons, Inc. Published 2024 by John Wiley & Sons, Inc.

INTRODUCTION

In the United States, older adults are becoming more racially diverse (American Community Survey, 2020), with an increasing proportion who are immigrants (Monserud, 2021). As populations age, racial and ethnic disparities in cognitive aging and in Alzheimer's disease and Alzheimer's disease-related dementias (AD/ADRD) are becoming more apparent, with research consistently showing that non-Hispanic Black (Black) and Hispanic (Latine) older adults perform worse on cognitive function tests and have higher risk for incidence of dementia than non-Hispanic White (White) older adults (Chen et al., 2022; Glymour & Manly, 2008; Mayeda et al., 2016; Weuve et al., 2018). Although less studied, immigrants may also have poorer baseline cognition and greater cognitive decline than non-immigrants (Kovaleva et al., 2021; Xu et al., 2017). Immigrants are more likely to have undiagnosed dementia compared to non-immigrants (Franco & Choi, 2020).

While common conceptions of racism focus on explicit experiences of stereotypes, prejudice, and discrimination, Critical Race Theory articulates how racism is also implicitly embedded in our societal structures and social dynamics (Ford & Airhihenbuwa, 2010). Critical Race Theory states that White supremacy encompasses the political, economic, social, and cultural systems that grant White people disproportionate power, resources, and opportunities over non-White racial and ethnic groups (Rollock & Gillborn, 2011). Following from these ideas, structural or systemic racism refers to how society's structures and systems codify racial differences to create inequitable access to power, resources, and opportunities for non-White racial and ethnic groups, including immigrants (Bailey et al., 2017; Misra et al., 2021; Rollock & Gillborn, 2011; Williams et al., 2019). In particular, structural racism encompasses the simultaneous and mutually reinforcing impacts of historical and current governmental and institutional policies across domains such as education, employment, health care, economic systems including credit, neighborhood residential segregation and housing markets, and the criminal legal system (Bailey et al., 2019; Williams et al., 2019). Much, but not all, of the impact of structural racism occurs via constrained educational and economic opportunities that lead to lower socioeconomic status (Phelan & Link, 2015). Importantly, structural racism also perpetuates an environment that condones interpersonal discrimination and stigma.

Structural racism likely influences cognitive aging through behavioral, physiological, psychosocial, and biological pathways. For example, structural racism may lead to fewer opportunities for high quality education and commensurate occupational opportunities, limited access to material and health care resources, as well as increased exposure to neighborhood disadvantage, individual discrimination, and other psychosocial stressors. Cumulative exposure to disadvantages resulting from structural racism may adversely affect one's physical and cognitive health through wear and tear on the body (Forrester et al., 2019; Geronimus, 1992).

In this chapter, we build on the introduction to the social determinants of health (SDOH) presented in the previous chapter to focus on how structural racism, discrimination, and stigma contribute to cognitive aging and AD/ADRD disparities for racial and ethnic minoritized people and immigrants through several key SDOH domains including racial residential segregation, neighborhood disadvantage, education, occupation, access to health care, and mass incarceration. Further, we discuss how clinical and research systems also perpetuate disparities via racial bias in cognitive assessment and diagnosis and

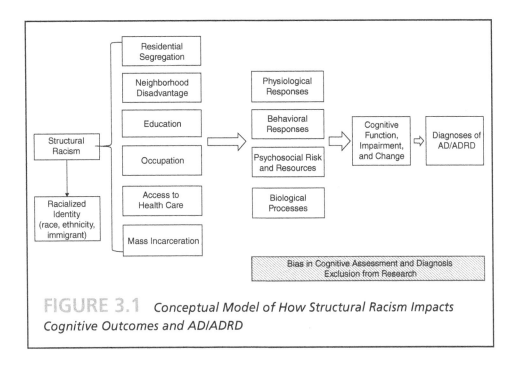

FIGURE 3.1 *Conceptual Model of How Structural Racism Impacts Cognitive Outcomes and AD/ADRD*

underrepresentation in research, and how this inaccurate and incomplete data is itself a form of structural racism. Finally, we consider how structural racism shapes racial discrimination and intersects with stigma around cognitive aging and AD/ADRD (Figure 3.1).

Racial Residential Segregation and Neighborhood Disadvantage

Structural racism contributes significantly to neighborhood-level disadvantage for racial and ethnic minoritized groups due to the historical and ongoing consequences of racial residential segregation, a system of physically separating Black and White racial groups that has been formally and informally reinforced through legislation and policies (Williams & Collins, 2001). Racial residential segregation has been identified as a fundamental cause of racial disparities, in large part because it has resulted in many low-income communities of color living in disinvested neighborhoods with fewer economic and social resources and greater exposure to environmental hazards like air pollution (Williams & Collins, 2001). For some non-Black communities of color, particularly immigrants, living in "ethnic enclaves" has often been considered protective because these neighborhoods offer greater access to social and community resources. However, the actual findings are mixed, as these communities often co-occur with concentrated poverty in disinvested neighborhoods (Bécares et al., 2012).

Current data are inconclusive about the impact of living in racially segregated neighborhoods on racial disparities in cognitive functioning. These studies primarily focus on current neighborhood composition and isolation, adjusting for individual and/or neighborhood economic conditions when possible. Two studies of Black racial segregation at either the neighborhood or metropolitan level found lower cognitive function among older adults with less than a high school education but no racial differences; the second study also did not find differences in cognitive decline over time (Aneshensel et al., 2011; Jang et al., 2022). In another study, living in Latine but not Black neighborhoods and counties was associated with better cognitive function at baseline but also greater cognitive decline over time for all older adults (Kovalchik et al., 2015), while still another study found the opposite: living in Black or Latine neighborhoods was associated with lower baseline cognitive function on some outcomes for Black and Latine older adults but also slower cognitive decline for Latine and White older adults (Meyer et al., 2021). There is a dearth of research describing the effects of living in an ethnic enclave on cognitive function among Asian American, Native Hawaiian and Pacific Islander (NH/PI) and American Indian and Alaskan Native (AI/AN) people, but at least one study suggested that among Chinese people in Chicago, living in an ethnic enclave may be a risk factor for poor cognitive outcomes (Guo et al., 2022). Only one study has looked at incident dementia among communities of color. This study found that the impact of racial segregation was most prominent among Black older adults for cognitive function followed by risk of dementia and more modest among Latine older adults (Pohl et al., 2021). No studies have assessed early life residential segregation on the cognitive function of older adults, even though anyone born before 1965 (i.e., over age 55) was exposed to Jim Crow laws that enforced racial segregation (Krieger et al., 2003). However, one study on school segregation earlier in life among Black older adults found that those who only attended segregated schools, compared to those who transitioned to integrated schools, had worse cognitive function (Peterson, George et al., 2021). Studies from the "Stroke Belt," a region of the southeastern United States with a high proportion of Black residents and history of slavery and subsequent Jim Crow laws, also provide insights. Black individuals born in the Stroke Belt have worse late-life cognitive function than those born elsewhere, even if they later move elsewhere; adjusting for early life SES and cardiovascular risk factors attenuate but do not completely explain the association between Stroke Belt birth and cognitive function (George et al., 2021).

More studies have looked at neighborhood disadvantage broadly, consistently finding associations with lower baseline cognitive function and greater cognitive decline over time, especially for individuals with lower socioeconomic status (Besser et al., 2021). Emerging research has also found associations with markers of AD/ADRD; for example, an autopsy study using brain bank data found that living in a disadvantaged neighborhood at the time of death was associated with an increased risk of AD neuropathology (Powell et al., 2020). Two longitudinal studies among Mexican American older adults found that neighborhood socioeconomic disadvantage was associated with cognitive function, after adjusting for socioeconomic status: one study found worse baseline cognitive function but not cognitive decline among their sample (Zeki Al Hazzouri et al., 2011) while the other study documented greater cognitive decline in their sample (Sheffield & Peek, 2009). However, the majority of the studies on neighborhood disadvantage has not investigated the potential impact of this factor on racial disparities, nor has this research focused explicitly on racial and ethnic minoritized or immigrant groups. To date, most neighborhood studies have been cross-sectional in design, with a potential for bias due to self-selection and reverse causation that warrant greater consideration in the future (Besser et al., 2021).

Segregated and disadvantaged neighborhoods are also associated with increased exposure to environmental risk factors. There is moderate to weak evidence that a select number of environmental risk factors contribute to risk of dementia (Killin et al., 2016), with the most robust, but still somewhat mixed, evidence pertaining to the potential contribution of air pollution, as measured by particulate fine matter (Peters et al., 2019; Weuve et al., 2021). However, almost no studies have considered whether environmental risk factors might help explain racial disparities in AD/ADRD. One longitudinal study of older women found that increased exposure to ambient fine particulate matter partially explained Black–White disparities in AD, and that Black women were around twice as likely to experience the adverse effects on risk of AD (Younan et al., 2021).

Education Quality, Literacy, and Years

Educational achievement gaps between White people and racial and ethnic minoritized groups have persisted for decades. In 2022, 45.5% of White people aged 25–29 had a bachelor's or higher degree, compared to 28.3% of Black people, 25.0% of Latine people, 28.4% of NH/PI people, and 11.8% of AI/AN people (US Census Bureau, 2022). These disparities, while narrowing somewhat over time, remain considerable. Structural racism has been acknowledged as a main contributor to educational achievement gaps across different racial and ethnic groups in the United States (Merolla & Jackson, 2019). Access to quality education, for example, is tied to housing policy, which has historically denied Black people and other minority groups equitable housing opportunities. Although some of the housing policies that mandated segregation in the past (e.g., redlining and Jim Crow laws) have now been banned, their negative impacts on racial and ethnic minoritized students' academic achievement and health outcomes persist today.

Among various modifiable social and behavioral factors, education provides the strongest explanation for racial disparities in cognitive function (Cagney & Lauderdale, 2002; Evans et al., 1997; Lövdén et al., 2020; Peterson et al., 2020). Structural racism results in school segregation and limited access to high-quality education, both of which contribute to racial disparities in cognitive outcomes among older populations. One recent study examined data from the Study of Healthy Aging in African Americans and found that Black individuals who attended integrated schools early in life had higher executive function and semantic memory than those who did not have any integrated school experience, suggesting that school segregation may be associated with worse cognitive outcomes in later life (Peterson, George et al., 2021). In another study using data from the Washington Heights-Inwood Columbia Aging Project, Sisco and colleagues assessed educational quality using six indicators of early life education quality, including the percentage of White students in the primary school that participants attended (i.e., a marker of segregated schools), urban versus rural location of the primary school, and whether the primary school had a single room for all grades. They found that educational quality explained 29% of the disparities in cognitive functioning, 26% in memory, and 32% in executive functioning (Sisco et al., 2015). Other studies using literacy (e.g., reading levels) as a proxy for quality of education have found that adjusting for literacy significantly attenuated racial disparities in cognitive function and dementia risk (Mehta et al., 2004; Yaffe et al., 2013).

Despite the important roles of school segregation and education quality in racial disparities in cognitive outcomes, most research has only assessed years of education. These studies have consistently shown that years of education explain racial disparities in cognitive function and AD/ADRD risk (Peterson et al., 2020; Weuve et al., 2018; Zahodne et al., 2017, 2021). Years of education accounted for around 20% of the relationship between race and cognition in a study using data from the National Social Life Health and Aging Project (Peterson et al., 2021). Another study, which used data from the Chicago Health and Aging Project, showed that years of education explained 35% of the Black–White disparities in performance of cognitive function tests (Weuve et al., 2018). Years of education may also explain racial disparities in incidence of dementia. One study found that Black–White disparities in dementia was sustainably attenuated after controlling for years of education and literacy levels (Yaffe et al., 2013).

Occupational Complexity, Occupational Hazards, and Job Strain

Structural racism also manifests as occupational segregation and discrimination against racial and ethnic minoritized workers. Minoritized and immigrant workers have historically faced higher unemployment rates and fewer job opportunities. Even when employed, they are more likely to be hired for jobs that are not commensurate with their education (De Jong & Madamba, 2001). Furthermore, minoritized and immigrant workers are more likely to be employed in jobs with lower pay, greater insecurity, fewer benefits, longer hours, and more occupational hazards (Misra et al., 2021; Steege et al., 2014).

Being employed in jobs with more occupational complexity has been linked to better cognitive performance later in life (Kaup et al., 2018; Lane et al., 2017; Sörman et al., 2019). According to the cognitive reserve theory, engaging in cognitively stimulating activities increases neuronal capacity, allowing the brain to compensate for neuronal damage that might manifest clinically as AD/ADRD (Stern, 2002). Occupational complexities are thought to contribute to cognitive reserve (Boots et al., 2015). Working in a complex environment allows people to exercise cognitive skills, stimulate intellectual abilities, and thus enhance cognitive functioning into old age. Due to disparities in access to high-skilled jobs, compared with White workers, minoritized and immigrant workers have fewer opportunities in their midlife to practice cognitive skills, which may contribute to poorer cognitive function as they age. Despite the potential role of occupational complexity in disparities in cognitive aging, only one study has investigated the roles of occupational complexity in disparities in cognitive aging. That study, which examined data from 7,357 Black and White participants aged 45 years and older, showed that occupational complexity explained a smaller proportion of the educational differences in cognitive function among Black men than it did among White men (Fujishiro et al., 2019).

Structural racism may also influence racial disparities in cognitive outcomes through differential exposure to occupational hazards. Research has shown that Black and Latine workers disproportionally work in segregated, dangerous, and toxic environments that present greater health and safety risks than White workers (Steege et al., 2014). As occupational hazards have been shown to cumulatively influence cognitive aging later in life (Gow et al., 2014), greater exposure to toxic work environments among minoritized and immigrant populations may result in disparities in cognitive function and dementia risk. However, little research has been conducted to investigate how work-related environmental hazards contribute to racial disparities in cognitive function.

Due to structural racism and discrimination in the workplace, racial and ethnic minoritized workers are also exposed to a higher level of job strain. A study of Black and White workers at four nursing homes in Massachusetts found that compared with White workers, Black workers on average worked seven more hours per week and earned $2.58 less per hour.

Furthermore, compared with White workers, Black workers were more likely to report high levels of job strain (Hurtado et al., 2012). Job strain has been linked to adverse cognitive outcomes from many large population cohort studies (Dong et al., 2018; Nilsen et al., 2021). However, we are unaware of any studies that have examined how disparities in job strain during adulthood may contribute to racial disparities in cognitive outcomes later in life.

Inequitable Access to Health Care

Compared with White individuals, racial and ethnic minoritized individual tend to receive dementia diagnostic services late in the illness, and once diagnosed, they are less likely to access antidementia treatment, trials, and care (Cooper et al., 2010; Tsoy et al., 2021). Residential segregation may result in limited access to quality care in minoritized communities. Higher concentrations of Black people have been associated with fewer primary care physicians (Gaskin et al., 2012). Providers treating Black patients are less likely to be board-certified and are more likely to report difficulty getting their patients to access to high-quality subspecialists, high-quality imaging, and non-emergency admission to the hospital (Bach et al., 2004). Lack of access to high-quality care in minoritized communities and underuse of specific AD/ADRD interventions may exacerbate the existing large racial disparities in cognitive outcomes. For instance, one study found that only 21% of American Indian and Alaskan Native people with dementia were medicated, a proportion that is substantially lower than the national figure of 49% of people with dementia being medicated (Avey et al., 2022). Additionally, research has shown increased caregiver burden for racial and ethnic minoritized adults with cognitive impairment, with non-White caregivers for persons with dementia reported having more unmet needs than White caregivers (Black et al., 2019).

Implicit bias and discrimination against racial and ethnic minoritized patients in health care settings may lead to reduced access to dementia care in these communities. In a survey of US caregivers of adults 50 or older with cognitive issues, more than a third of Black people and about a fifth of Latine and Asian people believed discrimination would be a barrier to receiving Alzheimer's care. Furthermore, more than half of the non-White adults reported experiencing discrimination when navigating health care settings for their care recipients (Alzheimer's Association, 2021). Discrimination in health care settings contributes to distrust of health care providers and reduces the likelihood of seeking appropriate dementia care when needed.

Mass Incarceration and the Aging Prison Population

Modern day structural racism is clearly exemplified in the mass incarceration of Black people, who experience harsher treatment at every stage of the criminal legal system and are incarcerated at five times the rates of White people in the United States (Bailey et al., 2021). Older adults are the largest growing population in prisons and growing at a faster rate than older adults in the general US population (Cipriani et al., 2017). People experiencing incarceration undergo an accelerated aging process that has led to a higher prevalence of chronic conditions at earlier ages and potential higher risk of developing dementia, including at earlier ages (Brooke et al., 2020). However, routine screening processes for cognitive function do not exist in prisons and the prevalence of dementia among older adults experiencing incarceration has not been firmly established. Available data indicate cognitive impairment is common among older adults who are incarcerated and are suggestive of a higher prevalence of dementia in prison settings compared to community settings (Brooke et al., 2020; Di Lorito et al., 2018; Peacock et al., 2019). It is highly likely that racial disparities in cognitive function are perpetuated within the carceral system, not only due to higher rates of incarceration but also higher prevalence of known risk factors preceding and during incarceration such as low educational attainment, psychiatric comorbidities, and traumatic brain injuries (Brooke et al., 2020). Emerging data also suggest higher risk of cognitive impairment and AD in older adults after being released from prisons (Kuffel et al., 2021). There is an urgent need to understand racial disparities in AD/ADRD for older adults experiencing incarceration, with careful consideration of ethical issues (Moore & Burtonwood, 2019) including whether screening tools developed in community settings might over- or underestimate cognitive problems among Black people in prison settings (Perez et al., 2021).

Structural Bias in Cognitive Assessment and Diagnosis

It has been suggested that clinical screening tools may not be as reliable for assessing cognitive impairment and dementia in racial and ethnic minoritized populations as they are in White populations (Fillenbaum et al., 1990). The Mini-Mental State Examination, for example, has been demonstrated to have particularly low specificity for Black community-dwelling adults, which could lead to more false positives of cognitive impairment among the Black population (Wood et al., 2006). In a study that linked medical claims data with the Health and Retirement Study participants aged 70 and older, Black participants were twice as likely as White participants to be underdiagnosed (Gianattasio et al., 2019). Misdiagnosis of dementia among racial and ethnic minoritized populations is likely caused by many screening tools being developed for White populations without accounting for cultural and linguistic differences between White people and racial and ethnic minoritized groups.

Structural racism for non-native and bilingual English speakers also manifests via the default language of cognitive assessments (i.e., English in the United States), which likely yields biased results for some racial and ethnic minoritized groups, particularly immigrants. Multiple studies have found that immigrants who have better acquisition of the language of the host country show better cognitive function (Xu et al., 2017). Meanwhile, limited English proficiency appears to help explain the higher rates of dementia – including undiagnosed dementia – among immigrants (Franco & Choi, 2020). These findings could reflect true differences in cognitive function and/or measurement issues in accurately capturing cognitive function. In addition to language proficiency, bilingualism could also impact cognitive assessments, with potential advantages in executive tasks and disadvantages in language-based tasks (Celik et al., 2022). To accurately assess cognitive function among populations with a wider variety of languages, cognitive tests should be translated into preferred languages, and cross-cultural and cross-linguistic reliability and validity should be established.

Clinical Research Exclusion Undergirded by Structural Racism

The impact of structural racism on AD/ADRD is represented within the research apparatus itself, both in terms of research prioritization and research participation. The dominant biomedical model has commonly assumed cognitive function and dementia can be fully understood via biological factors; however, it is becoming increasingly apparent that these findings are not generalizable to all populations. Although race is a social construct with no biological underpinnings, emerging research shows some racial and ethnic differences in AD/ADRD biomarkers and pathophysiology that warrant further study (Barnes, 2019).

Underrepresentation in AD/ADRD research is well-documented for racial and ethnic minoritized groups, those of lower socioeconomic status, and those living in rural areas (Gilmore-Bykovskyi et al., 2019; Indorewalla et al., 2021). A recent study also found underrepresentation of the most disadvantaged neighborhoods despite evidence that residents in those neighborhoods have higher risk for AD/ADRD (Grill et al., 2022). Dementia research commonly utilizes cohort studies, patient registries, and brain banks that rely on voluntary participant recruitment and retention. Structural racism undergirds this research underrepresentation via lack of trust of health care and research systems among communities of color due to such reasons as the well-documented history of unethical harm these systems have inflicted upon communities of color, language barriers including explicit exclusion of non-English speakers, accessibility and logistics challenges (e.g., costs, geography, requirement of a study partner), lower health literacy about AD/ADRD in particular and research more broadly, and lack of sufficient personnel, training, and resources dedicated to recruiting underrepresented populations (Gilmore-Bykovskyi et al., 2019; Indorewalla et al., 2021). Increasing efforts to recruit diverse older adults primarily focus on Black and Latine participants; other groups, including American Indians (AI), Alaska Natives (AN), NH/PI, those of lower socioeconomic status, and those from rural areas remain missing (Gilmore-Bykovskyi et al., 2019; Indorewalla et al., 2021). For example, efforts to expand clinical research to encompass Asian American and NH/PI communities may neglect to tailor materials and strategies to the linguistic and cultural specifics of diverse PI groups due to their small population sizes (Ta Park et al., 2021). When racial and ethnic minoritized people are recruited, structural inequities also exist through disproportionate exclusion during screening, such as for preexisting medical and/or psychiatric comorbidities (Indorewalla et al., 2021) or via cognitive screening using standardized eligibility criteria (Raman et al., 2021). Without accurate and representative data on cognitive function and AD/ADRD among these communities, it will be impossible to eliminate the resulting inequities.

Individual-Level Perceived Discrimination

Perceived discrimination is common among racial and ethnic minoritized individuals and has been shown to predict various health outcomes, including hypertension, diabetes, and mental disorders (MacGregor et al., 2020; Sims et al., 2012; Williams et al., 2012). Discrimination may lead to raised physiological responses such as increased blood pressure and heart rate, both of which are associated with lower levels of cognitive function and an increased risk for AD/ADRD. Additionally, discrimination may lead to the adoption of unhealthy behaviors, including smoking and drinking alcohol, as coping mechanisms for stress. Furthermore, as mentioned above, workplace discrimination may hinder workers from accessing jobs with high occupational complexity that could help maintain or improve cognitive performance.

A growing but limited body of research has investigated the association between perceived discrimination and cognitive outcomes, but the findings have been inconclusive. Barnes et al. used data from a cohort of 407 Black older adults without dementia and found that perceived discrimination was associated with poorer performance on cognitive function tests (Barnes et al., 2012). Similar findings were observed in the Midlife Development in the United States Study where perceived discrimination was associated with lower levels of cognitive function among middle-aged and older adults (Zahodne et al., 2017). However, in another study using data from 7,622 participants from the Health and Retirement Study, perceived discrimination was unrelated to cognitive function (Sutin et al., 2015). In a recent study of 1,712 adults from the Kaiser Healthy Aging and Diverse Life Experiences, everyday discrimination was not associated with cognitive function, while major lifetime discrimination was associated with better cognitive function scores among Black adults but not among other racial and ethnic groups (Meza et al., 2022). Several factors might account for the contradictory results, including differences in analytical approaches, populations, and measures of discrimination (e.g., everyday discrimination versus major lifetime discrimination).

The inconsistent findings on discrimination and cognitive function make it hard to draw meaningful conclusions about their relationship. Furthermore, these findings reveal the complexity and challenges of studying discrimination and cognitive function. Most studies examining discrimination and cognitive function are subject to selection bias. People who have experienced discrimination or have poorer cognitive outcomes are less likely to participate in a research study. As a result, the way in which participants are selected for a study may lead to collider bias, resulting in spurious links between discrimination and cognition. A second challenge with the study of discrimination and cognitive function concerns recall bias. In most studies, perceived discrimination was measured using a self-report scale administered retrospectively. Poor cognitive function may make it difficult for individuals to recall past discriminatory events, resulting in recall bias. This issue is especially problematic in cross-sectional studies in which perceived discrimination and cognitive function are measured simultaneously. In addition, discriminatory experiences vary by context, population, time, and place. Because most extant studies have examined perceived discrimination only among Black and White populations, we know very little about how discrimination is associated with cognitive function among Latine and Asian populations.

Stigma of Cognitive Aging and Dementia

Stigma refers to the negative beliefs and attitudes about and behaviors toward cognitive aging and AD/ADRD experienced by people with these conditions and their families. Stigma for AD/ADRD is common, and can have a profound impact on people's lives, including low self-esteem, social isolation, poor mental health, and decreased quality of life, as well as delaying diagnosis and deterring use of services (Nguyen & Li, 2020; Rosin et al., 2020). The aging process is already stigmatized. Limited understanding of what dementia is and how it differs from normal aging can increase stigma, particularly as dementia and AD are often conflated. However, an AD/ADRD diagnosis can also increase stigma as the lack of a treatment or cure is seen as a death sentence. It has been further suggested that emerging strategies for early detection (e.g., relying on mild cognitive impairment or preclinical/asymptomatic biomarkers) prior to a diagnosis might also activate this stigma (Rosin et al., 2020). For racial and ethnic minoritized and immigrant communities, stigma may be particularly harsh, although studies are limited. Some reasons for the greater impact among communities of color include lack of knowledge about AD/ADRD and cultural differences in expectations for healthy aging; specifically, early signs of dementia are often seen as a "normal" part of aging in ethnically diverse communities (Herrmann et al., 2018).

SUMMARY

Racial and ethnic disparities in cognitive function and AD/ADRD are well-established. Structural racism encompasses the totality of ways in which political, economic, social, and cultural systems create systemic disadvantage for racial and ethnic minoritized and immigrant groups, which then influence exposure to more commonly studied environmental, social, cultural, behavioral, and biological risk factors. We described how structural racism, in large part through racial residential segregation and constrained socioeconomic opportunities, contributes to disparities in neighborhood resources, environmental hazards, educational quality, occupational complexity, and access to health care that are linked to worse cognitive outcomes and AD/ADRD. However, research findings are often mixed due to an overall lack of studies on this topic and the substantial methodological limitations that plague extant studies. We highlighted the gap in data on disparities in the criminal legal system, within which there is a growing older population with no validated and routine screening processes. We also discussed how structural racism plays out in the clinical and research processes through racial bias in cognitive assessment and diagnosis and systemic exclusion from research, such that racial and ethnic minoritized and immigrant groups are severely under-represented in our existing knowledge base related to cognitive aging and AD/ADRD. We described how perceived racial discrimination also has mixed findings due to methodological limitations. Finally, we described how stigma associated with aging and dementia can further contribute to differential treatment of people living with AD/ADRD and their families.

Research on the impact of structural racism, discrimination, and stigma on cognitive aging and AD/ADRD is still in its infancy, with limited research across all major racial and ethnic groups including Black, Latine, Asian, NH/PI, and AI/AN populations and with limited inclusion of immigration status. Methodological challenges also persist, not only in measuring structural racism and cognition function and including representative samples, but also in addressing bias (e.g., selection bias), thus preventing us from establishing causal relationships between structural racism, discrimination, and cognitive function.

DISCUSSION QUESTIONS

1. What are some of the major challenges in measuring the impact of structural racism on cognitive function and AD/ADRD?

2. What are some potential structural strategies to improve cognitive assessment and research inclusion for racial and ethnic minoritized and immigrant groups?

3. How do you think racism and stigma might intersect for racial and ethnic minoritized and immigrant groups who experience cognitive impairment or dementia?

REFERENCES

Alzheimer's Association. (2021). *2021 Alzheimer's Disease Facts and Figures.* https://www.alz.org/media/documents/alzheimers-facts-and-figures.pdf

American Community Survey. (2020). *American Community Survey.* https://www.census.gov/programs-surveys/acs

Aneshensel, C. S., Ko, M. J., Chodosh, J., & Wight, R. G. (2011). The urban neighborhood and cognitive functioning in late middle age. *Journal of Health and Social Behavior, 52*(2), 163–179. https://doi.org/10.1177/0022146510393974

Avey, J. P., Schaefer, K. R., Noonan, C. J., Muller, C. J., Mosley, M., & Galvin, J. E. (2022). Patterns of healthcare use and mortality after Alzheimer's disease or related Dementia diagnosis among alaska native patients: Results of a cluster analysis in a tribal healthcare setting. *Journal of Alzheimer's Disease Reports*, 6(1), 401–410. https://doi.org/10.3233/ADR-210062

Bach, P. B., Pham, H. H., Schrag, D., Tate, R. C., & Hargraves, J. L. (2004). Primary care physicians who treat blacks and whites. *New England Journal of Medicine*, 351(6), 575–584. https://doi.org/10.1056/NEJMsa040609

Bailey, Z. D., Feldman, J. M., & Bassett, M. T. (2021). *How structural racism works—Racist policies as a root cause of US racial health inequities*. Mass Medical Soc.

Bailey, Z. D., Krieger, N., Agénor, M., Graves, J., Linos, N., & Bassett, M. T. (2017). Structural racism and health inequities in the USA: Evidence and interventions. *The Lancet*, 389(10077), 1453–1463. https://doi.org/10.1016/S0140-6736(17)30569-X

Bailey, Z. D., Krieger, N., Agénor, M., Graves, J., Linos, N., & Bassett, M. T. (2019). Structural racism and health inequities in the United States of America: Evidence and interventions. In Jonathan Oberlander, Mara Buchbinder, Larry R. Churchill, Sue E. Estroff, Nancy M. P. King, Barry F. Saunders, Ronald P. Strauss, Rebecca L. Walker *The social medicine reader, Volume II, Third Edition* (pp. 209–234). Duke University Press. https://www.dukeupress.edu/the-social-medicine-reader-third-edition-volume-two https://www.dukeupress.edu/the-social-medicine-reader-third-edition-volume-two

Barnes, L. L. (2019). Biomarkers for Alzheimer dementia in diverse racial and ethnic minorities—A public health priority. *JAMA Neurology*, 76(3), 251–253. https://doi.org/10.1001/jamaneurol.2018.3444

Barnes, L. L., Lewis, T. T., Begeny, C. T., Yu, L., Bennett, D. A., & Wilson, R. S. (2012). Perceived discrimination and cognition in older African Americans. *Journal of the International Neuropsychological Society*, 18(5), 856–865. https://doi.org/10.1017/S1355617712000628

Bécares, L., Nazroo, J., Albor, C., Chandola, T., & Stafford, M. (2012). Examining the differential association between self-rated health and area deprivation among white British and ethnic minority people in England. *Social Science & Medicine*, 74(4), 616–624. https://doi.org/10.1016/j.socscimed.2011.11.007

Besser, L. M., Brenowitz, W. D., Meyer, O. L., Hoermann, S., & Renne, J. (2021). Methods to address self-selection and reverse causation in studies of neighborhood environments and brain health. *International Journal of Environmental Research and Public Health*, 18(12), 6484. https://doi.org/10.3390/ijerph18126484

Black, B. S., Johnston, D., Leoutsakos, J., Reuland, M., Kelly, J., Amjad, H., Davis, K., Willink, A., Sloan, D., & Lyketsos, C. (2019). Unmet needs in community-living persons with dementia are common, often non-medical and related to patient and caregiver characteristics. *International Psychogeriatrics*, 31(11), 1643–1654. https://doi.org/10.1017/S1041610218002296

Boots, E. A., Schultz, S. A., Almeida, R. P., Oh, J. M., Koscik, R. L., Dowling, M. N., Gallagher, C. L., Carlsson, C. M., Rowley, H. A., & Bendlin, B. B. (2015). Occupational complexity and cognitive reserve in a middle-aged cohort at risk for Alzheimer's disease. *Archives of Clinical Neuropsychology*, 30(7), 634–642. https://doi.org/10.1093/arclin/acv041

Brooke, J., Diaz-Gil, A., & Jackson, D. (2020). The impact of dementia in the prison setting: A systematic review. *Dementia*, 19(5), 1509–1531. https://doi.org/10.1177/1471301218801715

Cagney, K. A., & Lauderdale, D. S. (2002). Education, wealth, and cognitive function in later life. *The Journals of Gerontology Series B: Psychological Sciences and Social Sciences*, 57(2), 163–P172. https://doi.org/10.1093/geronb/57.2.p163

Celik, S., Kokje, E., Meyer, P., Frölich, L., & Teichmann, B. (2022). Does bilingualism influence neuropsychological test performance in older adults? A systematic review. *Applied Neuropsychology: Adult*, 29(4), 855–873. https://doi.org/10.1080/23279095.2020.1788032

Chen, R., Weuve, J., Misra, S., Cuevas, A., Kubzansky, L. D., & Williams, D. R. (2022). Racial disparities in cognitive function among middle-aged and older adults: The roles of cumulative stress exposures across the life course. *The Journals of Gerontology: Series A. Biological Sciences and Medical Sciences*, 77(2), 357–364. https://doi.org/10.1093/gerona/glab099

Chen, R., Weuve, J., Misra, S., Cuevas, A., Kubzansky, L. D., & Williams, D. R. (2022). Racial disparities in cognitive function among middle-aged and older adults: The roles of cumulative stress exposures across the life course. *The Journals of Gerontology: Series A.*

Cipriani, G., Danti, S., Carlesi, C., & Di Fiorino, M. (2017). Old and dangerous: Prison and dementia. *Journal of Forensic and Legal Medicine*, 51, 40–44. https://doi.org/10.1016/j.jflm.2017.07.004

Cooper, C., Tandy, A. R., Balamurali, T. B., & Livingston, G. (2010). A systematic review and meta-analysis of ethnic differences in use of dementia treatment, care, and research. *The American Journal of Geriatric Psychiatry*, 18(3), 193–203. https://doi.org/10.1097/JGP.0b013e3181bf9caf

De Jong, G. F., & Madamba, A. B. (2001). A double disadvantage? Minority group, immigrant status, and underemployment in the United States. *Social Science Quarterly*, *82*(1), 117–130. https://doi.org/10.1111/0038-4941.00011

Di Lorito, C., Völlm, B., & Dening, T. (2018). Psychiatric disorders among older prisoners: A systematic review and comparison study against older people in the community. *Aging & Mental Health*, *22*(1), 1–10. https://doi.org/10.1080/13607863.2017.1286453

Dong, L., Eaton, W. W., Spira, A. P., Agnew, J., Surkan, P. J., & Mojtabai, R. (2018). Job strain and cognitive change: The Baltimore epidemiologic catchment area follow-up study. *Occupational and Environmental Medicine*, *75*(12), 856–862. https://doi.org/10.1136/oemed-2018-105213

Evans, D. A., Hebert, L. E., Beckett, L. A., Scherr, P. A., Albert, M. S., Chown, M. J., Pilgrim, D. M., & Taylor, J. O. (1997). Education and other measures of socioeconomic status and risk of incident Alzheimer disease in a defined population of older persons. *Archives of Neurology*, *54*(11), 1399–1405. https://doi.org/10.1001/archneur.1997.00550230066019

Fillenbaum, G., Heyman, A., Williams, K., Prosnitz, B., & Burchett, B. (1990). Sensitivity and specificity of standardized screens of cognitive impairment and dementia among elderly black and white community residents. *Journal of Clinical Epidemiology*, *43*(7), 651–660. https://doi.org/10.1016/0895-4356(90)90035-n

Ford, C. L., & Airhihenbuwa, C. O. (2010). Critical race theory, race equity, and public health: Toward antiracism praxis. *American Journal of Public Health*, *100*(S1), S30–S35. https://doi.org/10.2105/AJPH.2009.171058

Forrester, S. N., Gallo, J. J., Whitfield, K. E., & Thorpe, R. J., Jr. (2019). A framework of minority stress: From physiological manifestations to cognitive outcomes. *The Gerontologist*, *59*(6), 1017–1023. https://doi.org/10.1093/geront/gny104

Franco, Y., & Choi, E. Y. (2020). The relationship between immigrant status and undiagnosed dementia: The role of limited English proficiency. *Journal of Immigrant and Minority Health*, *22*(5), 914–922. https://doi.org/10.1007/s10903-019-00963-w

Fujishiro, K., MacDonald, L. A., Crowe, M., McClure, L. A., Howard, V. J., & Wadley, V. G. (2019). The role of occupation in explaining cognitive functioning in later life: Education and occupational complexity in a US national sample of black and white men and women. *The Journals of Gerontology: Series B*, *74*(7), 1189–1199. https://doi.org/10.1093/geronb/gbx112

Gaskin, D. J., Dinwiddie, G. Y., Chan, K. S., & McCleary, R. (2012). Residential segregation and disparities in health care services utilization. *Medical Care Research and Review*, *69*(2), 158–175. https://doi.org/10.1177/1077558711420263

George, K. M., Peterson, R. L., Gilsanz, P., Barnes, L. L., Mayeda, E. R., Glymour, M. M., Mungas, D. M., DeCarli, C. S., & Whitmer, R. A. (2021). Stroke belt birth state and late-life cognition in the study of healthy aging in African Americans (STAR). *Annals of Epidemiology*, *64*, 26–32. https://doi.org/10.1016/j.annepidem.2021.09.001

Geronimus, A. T. (1992). The weathering hypothesis and the health of African-American women and infants: Evidence and speculations. *Ethnicity & Disease*, *2*(3), 207–221.

Gianattasio, K. Z., Wu, Q., Glymour, M. M., & Power, M. C. (2019). Comparison of methods for algorithmic classification of dementia status in the health and retirement study. *Epidemiology (Cambridge, Mass.)*, *30*(2), 291. https://doi.org/10.1097/EDE.0000000000000945

Gilmore-Bykovskyi, A. L., Jin, Y., Gleason, C., Flowers-Benton, S., Block, L. M., Dilworth-Anderson, P., Barnes, L. L., Shah, M. N., & Zuelsdorff, M. (2019). Recruitment and retention of underrepresented populations in Alzheimer's disease research: A systematic review. *Alzheimer's & Dementia: Translational Research & Clinical Interventions*, *5*, 751–770. https://doi.org/10.1016/j.trci.2019.09.018

Glymour, M. M., & Manly, J. J. (2008). Lifecourse social conditions and racial and ethnic patterns of cognitive aging. *Neuropsychology Review*, *18*(3), 223–254. https://doi.org/10.1007/s11065-008-9064-z

Gow, A. J., Avlund, K., & Mortensen, E. L. (2014). Occupational characteristics and cognitive aging in the Glostrup 1914 Cohort. *Journals of Gerontology Series B: Psychological Sciences and Social Sciences*, *69*(2), 228–236. https://doi.org/10.1093/geronb/gbs115

Grill, J. D., Kind, A., Hoang, D., & Gillen, D. L. (2022). Diversifying Recruitment Registries: Considering Neighborhood Health Metrics. *The journal of prevention of Alzheimer's disease*, *9*(1), 119–125. https://doi.org/10.14283/jpad.2021.50

Guo, M., Wang, Y., Xu, H., Li, M., Wu, B., & Dong, X. (2022). Is living in an ethnic enclave associated with cognitive function? Results from the population study of Chinese elderly (PINE) in Chicago. *The Gerontologist*, *62*(5), 662–673. https://doi.org/10.1093/geront/gnab158

Herrmann, L. K., Welter, E., Leverenz, J., Lerner, A. J., Udelson, N., Kanetsky, C., & Sajatovic, M. (2018). A systematic review of dementia-related stigma research: Can we move the stigma dial? *The American Journal of Geriatric Psychiatry*, *26*(3), 316–331. https://doi.org/10.1016/j.jagp.2017.09.006

Hurtado, D. A., Sabbath, E. L., Ertel, K. A., Buxton, O. M., & Berkman, L. F. (2012). Racial disparities in job strain among American and immigrant long-term care workers. *International Nursing Review*, *59*(2), 237–244. https://doi.org/10.1111/j.1466-7657.2011.00948.x

Indorewalla, K. K., O'Connor, M. K., Budson, A. E., Guess DiTerlizzi, C., & Jackson, J. (2021). Modifiable barriers for recruitment and retention of older adults participants from underrepresented minorities in Alzheimer's disease research. *Journal of Alzheimer's disease : JAD*, *80*(3), 927–940. https://doi.org/10.3233/JAD-201081

Jang, J. B., Hicken, M. T., Mullins, M., Esposito, M., Sol, K., Manly, J. J., Judd, S., Wadley, V., & Clarke, P. J. (2022). Racial segregation and cognitive function among older adults in the United States: Findings from the reasons for geographic and racial differences in stroke study. *The Journals of Gerontology. Series B, Psychological Sciences and Social Sciences*, *77*(6), 1132–1143. https://doi.org/10.1093/geronb/gbab107

Kaup, A. R., Xia, F., Launer, L. J., Sidney, S., Nasrallah, I., Erus, G., Allen, N., & Yaffe, K. (2018). Occupational cognitive complexity in earlier adulthood is associated with brain structure and cognitive health in midlife: The CARDIA study. *Neuropsychology*, *32*(8), 895. https://doi.org/10.1037/neu0000474

Killin, L. O., Starr, J. M., Shiue, I. J., & Russ, T. C. (2016). Environmental risk factors for dementia: A systematic review. *BMC Geriatrics*, *16*(1), 1–28. https://doi.org/10.1186/s12877-016-0342-y

Kovalchik, S. A., Slaughter, M. E., Miles, J., Friedman, E. M., & Shih, R. A. (2015). Neighbourhood racial/ethnic composition and segregation and trajectories of cognitive decline among US older adults. *Journal of Epidemiology and Community Health*, *69*(10), 978–984. https://doi.org/10.1136/jech-2015-205600

Kovaleva, M., Jones, A., Maxwell, C. A., & Long, E. M. (2021). Immigrants and dementia: Literature update. *Geriatric Nursing*, *42*(5), 1218–1221. https://doi.org/10.1016/j.gerinurse.2021.04.019

Krieger, N., Waterman, P. D., Chen, J. T., Soobader, M. J., & Subramanian, S. V. (2003). Monitoring socioeconomic inequalities in sexually transmitted infections, tuberculosis, and violence: geocoding and choice of area-based socioeconomic measures--the public health disparities geocoding project (US). *Public Health Reports (Washington, D.C. : 1974)*, *118*(3), 240–260. https://doi.org/10.1093/phr/118.3.240

Kuffel, R., Byers, A., Williams, B., Fortinsky, R., Boscardin, J., Li, Y., & Barry, L. (2021). High occurrence of dementia in older adults returning to community from prison. *The American Journal of Geriatric Psychiatry*, *29*(4), S45–S47. https://doi.org/10.1093/geroni/igaa057.843

Lane, A. P., Windsor, T. D., Andel, R., & Luszcz, M. A. (2017). Is occupational complexity associated with cognitive performance or decline? Results from the Australian longitudinal study of ageing. *Gerontology*, *63*(6), 550–559. https://doi.org/10.1159/000475559

Lövdén, M., Fratiglioni, L., Glymour, M. M., Lindenberger, U., & Tucker-Drob, E. M. (2020). Education and cognitive functioning across the life span. *Psychological Science in the Public Interest*, *21*(1), 6–41. https://doi.org/10.1177/1529100620920576

MacGregor, C., Freedman, A., Keenan-Devlin, L., Grobman, W., Wadhwa, P., Simhan, H. N., Buss, C., & Borders, A. (2020). Maternal perceived discrimination and association with gestational diabetes. *American Journal of Obstetrics & Gynecology MFM*, *2*(4), 100222. https://doi.org/10.1016/j.ajogmf.2020.100222

Mayeda, E. R., Glymour, M. M., Quesenberry, C. P., & Whitmer, R. A. (2016). Inequalities in dementia incidence between six racial and ethnic groups over 14 years. *Alzheimer's & Dementia*, *12*(3), 216–224. https://doi.org/10.1016/j.jalz.2015.12.007

Mehta, K. M., Simonsick, E. M., Rooks, R., Newman, A. B., Pope, S. K., Rubin, S. M., Yaffe, K., Health, A., & Body Composition Study. (2004). Black and white differences in cognitive function test scores: What explains the difference? *Journal of the American Geriatrics Society*, *52*(12), 2120–2127. https://doi.org/10.1111/j.1532-5415.2004.52575.x

Merolla, D. M., & Jackson, O. (2019). Structural racism as the fundamental cause of the academic achievement gap. *Sociology Compass*, *13*(6), e12696. https://doi.org/10.1111/soc4.12696

Meyer, O. L., Besser, L., Mitsova, D., Booker, M., Luu, E., Tobias, M., Farias, S. T., Mungas, D., DeCarli, C., & Whitmer, R. A. (2021). Neighborhood racial/ethnic segregation and cognitive decline in older adults. *Social Science & Medicine*, *284*, 114226. https://doi.org/10.1016/j.socscimed.2021.114226

Meza, E., Peterson, R., Gilsanz, P., George, K. M., Miles, S. J., Eng, C. W., Mungas, D. M., Mayeda, E. R., Glymour, M. M., & Whitmer, R. A. (2022). Perceived discrimination, nativity, and cognitive performance in a multi-ethnic study of older adults: Findings from the Kaiser Healthy Aging and Diverse Life Experiences (KHANDLE) Study. *The Journals of Gerontology: Series A, Biological Sciences and Medical Sciences*, *77*(2), e65–e73. https://doi.org/10.1093/gerona/glab170

Misra, S., Kwon, S. C., Abraído-Lanza, A. F., Chebli, P., Trinh-Shevrin, C., & Yi, S. S. (2021). Structural racism and immigrant health in the United States. *Health Education & Behavior*, *48*(3), 332–341. https://doi.org/10.1177/10901981211010676

Monserud, M. A. (2021). Later-life trajectories of cognitive functioning among immigrants of Mexican origin: Implications of age at immigration and social resources. *Ethnicity & Health, 26*(5), 720–736. : https://doi.org/10.1080/13557858.2018.1547370

Moore, K. J., & Burtonwood, J. (2019). Are we failing to meet the healthcare needs of prisoners with dementia? *International Psychogeriatrics, 31*(8), 1071–1074. https://doi.org/10.1017/S104161021900108X

Nguyen, T., & Li, X. (2020). Understanding public-stigma and self-stigma in the context of dementia: A systematic review of the global literature. *Dementia, 19*(2), 148–181. https://doi.org/10.1177/1471301218800122

Nilsen, C., Nelson, M. E., Andel, R., Crowe, M., Finkel, D., & Pedersen, N. L. (2021). Job strain and trajectories of cognitive change before and after retirement. *The Journals of Gerontology: Series B B, Psychological Sciences and Social Sciences, 76*(7), 1313–1322. https://doi.org/10.1093/geronb/gbab033

Peacock, S., Burles, M., Hodson, A., Kumaran, M., MacRae, R., Peternelj-Taylor, C., & Holtslander, L. (2019). Older persons with dementia in prison: An integrative review. *International Journal of Prisoner Health. 16*(1), 1–16. https://doi.org/10.1108/IJPH-01-2019-0007

Perez, A., Manning, K. J., Powell, W., & Barry, L. C. (2021). Cognitive impairment in older incarcerated males: education and race considerations. *The American journal of geriatric psychiatry: official journal of the American Association for Geriatric Psychiatry, 29*(10), 1062–1073. https://doi.org/10.1016/j.jagp.2021.05.014

Peters, R., Ee, N., Peters, J., Booth, A., Mudway, I., & Anstey, K. J. (2019). Air pollution and dementia: A systematic review. *Journal of Alzheimer's Disease, 70*(s1), S145–S163. https://doi.org/10.3233/JAD-180631

Peterson, R. L., Butler, E. A., Ehiri, J. E., Fain, M. J., & Carvajal, S. C. (2021). Mechanisms of racial disparities in cognitive aging: An examination of material and psychosocial well-being. *The Journals of Gerontology: Series B, 76*(3), 574–582. https://doi.org/10.1093/geronb/gbaa003

Peterson, R. L., Fain, M. J., Butler, A., Ehiri, J. E., & Carvajal, S. C. (2020). The role of social and behavioral risk factors in explaining racial disparities in age-related cognitive impairment: A structured narrative review. *Aging, Neuropsychology, and Cognition, 27*(2), 173–196. https://doi.org/10.1080/13825585.2019.1598539

Peterson, R. L., George, K. M., Barnes, L. L., Gilsanz, P., Mayeda, E. R., Glymour, M. M., Mungas, D. M., & Whitmer, R. A. (2021). Association of timing of school desegregation in the United States with late-life cognition in the study of healthy aging in African Americans (STAR) cohort. *JAMA Network Open, 4*(10), e2129052–e2129052. https://doi.org/10.1001/jamanetworkopen.2021.29052

Phelan, J. C., & Link, B. G. (2015). Is racism a fundamental cause of inequalities in health? *Annual Review of Sociology, 41*, 311–330. https://doi.org/10.1146/annurev-soc-073014-112305

Pohl, D. J., Seblova, D., Avila, J. F., Dorsman, K. A., Kulick, E. R., Casey, J. A., & Manly, J. (2021). Relationship between residential segregation, later-life cognition, and incident Dementia across race/ethnicity. *International Journal of Environmental Research and Public Health, 18*(21), 11233. https://doi.org/10.3390/ijerph182111233

Powell, W. R., Buckingham, W. R., Larson, J. L., Vilen, L., Yu, M., Salamat, M. S., Bendlin, B. B., Rissman, R. A., & Kind, A. J. (2020). Association of neighborhood-level disadvantage with Alzheimer disease neuropathology. *JAMA Network Open, 3*(6), e207559–e207559. https://doi.org/10.1001/jamanetworkopen.2020.7559

Raman, R., Quiroz, Y. T., Langford, O., Choi, J., Ritchie, M., Baumgartner, M., Rentz, D., Aggarwal, N. T., Aisen, P., & Sperling, R. (2021). Disparities by race and ethnicity among adults recruited for a preclinical Alzheimer disease trial. *JAMA Network Open, 4*(7), e2114364–e2114364. https://doi.org/10.1001/jamanetworkopen.2021.14364

Rollock, N., & Gillborn, D. (2011). Critical race theory (CRT). *British Educational Research Association.*

Rosin, E. R., Blasco, D., Pilozzi, A. R., Yang, L. H., & Huang, X. (2020). A narrative review of Alzheimer's disease stigma. *Journal of Alzheimer's Disease, Preprint*, 1–14. https://doi.org/10.3233/JAD-200932

Sheffield, K. M., & Peek, M. K. (2009). Neighborhood context and cognitive decline in older Mexican Americans: Results from the hispanic established populations for epidemiologic studies of the elderly. *American Journal of Epidemiology, 169*(9), 1092–1101. https://doi.org/10.1093/aje/kwp005

Sims, M., Diez-Roux, A. V., Dudley, A., Gebreab, S., Wyatt, S. B., Bruce, M. A., James, S. A., Robinson, J. C., Williams, D. R., & Taylor, H. A. (2012). Perceived discrimination and hypertension among African Americans in the Jackson heart study. *American Journal of Public Health, 102*(S2), S258–S265. https://doi.org/10.2105/AJPH.2011.300523

Sisco, S., Gross, A. L., Shih, R. A., Sachs, B. C., Glymour, M. M., Bangen, K. J., Benitez, A., Skinner, J., Schneider, B. C., & Manly, J. J. (2015). The role of early-life educational quality and literacy in explaining racial disparities in cognition in late life. *Journals of Gerontology Series B: Psychological Sciences and Social Sciences, 70*(4), 557–567. https://doi.org/10.1093/geronb/gbt133

Sörman, D. E., Hansson, P., Pritschke, I., & Ljungberg, J. K. (2019). Complexity of primary lifetime occupation and cognitive processing. *Frontiers in Psychology, 10*, 1861. https://doi.org/10.3389/fpsyg.2019.01861

Steege, A. L., Baron, S. L., Marsh, S. M., Menéndez, C. C., & Myers, J. R. (2014). Examining occupational health and safety disparities using national data: A cause for continuing concern. *American Journal of Industrial Medicine*, *57*(5), 527–538. https://doi.org/10.1002/ajim.22297

Stern, Y. (2002). What is cognitive reserve? Theory and research application of the reserve concept. *Journal of the International Neuropsychological Society*, *8*(3), 448–460. https://doi.org/10.1017/s1355617702813248

Sutin, A. R., Stephan, Y., Carretta, H., & Terracciano, A. (2015). Perceived discrimination and physical, cognitive, and emotional health in older adulthood. *The American Journal of Geriatric Psychiatry*, *23*(2), 171–179. https://doi.org/10.1016/j.jagp.2014.03.007

Ta Park, V., Grill, J. D., Zhu, J., Nguyen, K., Nam, B., Tsoh, J., Kanaya, A., Vuong, Q., Bang, J., Nguyen, N. C. Y., Cho, I. H., Gallagher-Thompson, D., Hinton, L., & Meyer, O. L. (2021). Asian Americans and Pacific Islanders' perspectives on participating in the CARE recruitment research registry for Alzheimer's disease and related dementias, aging, and caregiving research. *Alzheimer's & Dementia (New York, N. Y.)*, *7*(1), e12195. https://doi.org/10.1002/trc2.12195

Tsoy, E., Kiekhofer, R. E., Guterman, E. L., Tee, B. L., Windon, C. C., Dorsman, K. A., Lanata, S. C., Rabinovici, G. D., Miller, B. L., Kind, A. J. H., & Possin, K. L. (2021). Assessment of Racial/Ethnic disparities in timeliness and comprehensiveness of dementia diagnosis in california. *JAMA Neurology*, *78*(6), 657–665. https://doi.org/10.1001/jamaneurol.2021.0399

U.S. Census Bureau. (2022 October). *Current Population Survey (CPS), Annual Social and Economic Supplement, 1970 through 2022*. Available at: https://www.census.gov/programs-surveys/cps.html

Weuve, J., Barnes, L. L., de Leon, C. F. M., Rajan, K. B., Beck, T., Aggarwal, N. T., Hebert, L. E., Bennett, D. A., Wilson, R. S., & Evans, D. A. (2018). Cognitive aging in black and white Americans: Cognition, cognitive decline, and incidence of Alzheimer disease dementia. *Epidemiology (Cambridge, Mass.)*, *29*(1), 151. https://doi.org/10.1097/EDE.0000000000000747

Weuve, J., Bennett, E. E., Ranker, L., Gianattasio, K. Z., Pedde, M., Adar, S. D., Yanosky, J. D., & Power, M. C. (2021). Exposure to air pollution in relation to risk of dementia and related outcomes: An updated systematic review of the epidemiological literature. *Environmental Health Perspectives*, *129*(9), 096001. https://doi.org/10.1289/EHP8716

Williams, D. R., & Collins, C. (2001). Racial residential segregation: A fundamental cause of racial disparities in health. *Public Health Reports (Washington, D.C. : 1974)*, *116*(5), 404–416. https://doi.org/10.1093/phr/116.5.404

Williams, D. R., Haile, R., Mohammed, S. A., Herman, A., Sonnega, J., Jackson, J. S., & Stein, D. J. (2012). Perceived discrimination and psychological well-being in the USA and South Africa. *Ethnicity & Health*, *17*(1–2), 111–133. https://doi.org/10.1080/13557858.2012.654770

Williams, D. R., Lawrence, J. A., & Davis, B. A. (2019). Racism and health: Evidence and needed research. *Annual Review of Public Health*, *40*, 105–125. https://doi.org/10.1146/annurev-publhealth-040218-043750

Wood, R. Y., Giuliano, K. K., Bignell, C. U., & Pritham, W. W. (2006). Assessing cognitive ability in research: Use of MMSE with minority populations and elderly adults with low education levels. *Journal of Gerontological Nursing*, *32*(4), 45–54. https://doi.org/10.3928/00989134-20060401-08

Xu, H., Zhang, Y., & Wu, B. (2017). Association between migration and cognitive status among middle-aged and older adults: A systematic review. *BMC Geriatrics*, *17*(1), 1–15. https://doi.org/10.1186/s12877-017-0585-2

Yaffe, K., Falvey, C., Harris, T. B., Newman, A., Satterfield, S., Koster, A., Ayonayon, H., & Simonsick, E. (2013). Effect of socioeconomic disparities on incidence of dementia among biracial older adults: Prospective study. *BMJ*, *347*, https://doi.org/10.1136/bmj.f7051

Younan, D., Wang, X., Gruenewald, T., Gatz, M., Serre, M. L., Vizuete, W., Braskie, M. N., Woods, N. F., Kahe, K., & Garcia, L. (2021). Racial/Ethnic disparities in Alzheimer's disease risk: Role of exposure to ambient fine particles. *The Journals of Gerontology: Series A*. https://doi.org/10.1093/gerona/glab231

Zahodne, L. B., Manly, J. J., Smith, J., Seeman, T., & Lachman, M. E. (2017). Socioeconomic, health, and psychosocial mediators of racial disparities in cognition in early, middle, and late adulthood. *Psychology and Aging*, *32*(2), 118. https://doi.org/10.1037/pag0000154

Zahodne, L. B., Sharifian, N., Kraal, A. Z., Zaheed, A. B., Sol, K., Morris, E. P., Schupf, N., Manly, J. J., & Brickman, A. M. (2021). Socioeconomic and psychosocial mechanisms underlying racial/ethnic disparities in cognition among older adults. *Neuropsychology*, *35*(3), 265. https://doi.org/10.1037/neu0000720

Zeki Al Hazzouri, A., Haan, M. N., Kalbfleisch, J. D., Galea, S., Lisabeth, L. D., & Aiello, A. E. (2011). Life-course socioeconomic position and incidence of dementia and cognitive impairment without dementia in older Mexican Americans: Results from the Sacramento area Latino study on aging. *American Journal of Epidemiology*, *173*(10), 1148–1158. https://doi.org/10.1093/aje/kwq483

CHAPTER

INTERSECTIONAL SYNDEMICS AND AGING AMONG LESBIAN, GAY, BISEXUAL, TRANSGENDER, AND QUEER (LGBTQ+) COMMUNITIES

OHSHUE GATANAGA, SAHNAH LIM

LEARNING OBJECTIVES

By the end of this chapter, readers will be able to:

- Explore the multiplicative impact of social identities (i.e., intersectionality) and implications on aging and Alzheimer's disease and Alzheimer's disease-related dementias (AD/ADRD) among people who are members of lesbian, gay, bisexual, transgender, queer, and other (LGBTQ+) communities as well as racial and ethnic minoritized, low income, and other vulnerable populations.

Population Science Methods and Approaches to Aging and Alzheimer's Disease and Related Dementias Research, First Edition. Edited by Chau Trinh-Shevrin.
© 2024 John Wiley & Sons, Inc. Published 2024 by John Wiley & Sons, Inc.

- Identify the co-occurring micro-, mezzo-, and macro-level psychosocial factors (i.e., syndemic factors) and policies that impact the care of older LGBTQ+ adults with dementia.
- Explore how an intersectional syndemics framework is useful in understanding the unique experiences of aging and AD/ADRD in LGBTQ+, racial and ethnic minoritized, and other vulnerable populations.

INTRODUCTION

Exploring aging and Alzheimer's disease and Alzheimer's disease-related dementias (AD/ADRD) within LGBTQ+ populations and other intersecting identities in the United States has only recently emerged as an area of interest in public health research – the result of changes in demographics and societal mores combined with a general growing interest in the health of the aging population.[1] Rapid demographic shifts are leading to a larger proportion of adults over 65 years old (Urban Institute, 2022), and within this population of older adults, there is a growing proportion of self-identified LGBTQ+ individuals (Jones, 2022). One reason for this change is that HIV/AIDS research and public health interventions have vastly improved the quality of life for LGBTQ+ individuals, who were and continue to be uniquely impacted by the AIDS pandemic. In addition, more older adults identify as LGBTQ+ than ever before, as self-identification has become increasingly acceptable within US society. In 2017, there were approximately 2.7 million LGBTQ+ adults over the age of 50 in the United States, as compared to 2.4 million in 2016 (Choi & Meyer, 2016; MAP, 2017). The number of LGBTQ+ adults is expected to grow rapidly over the next decades as Baby Boomers age, contributing to an increase in the older adult population overall, and shifts in social mores further facilitate and support LGBTQ+ self-identification (MAP, 2017).[2]

Research about LGBTQ+ people with dementia remains in its nascent stage (Kimmel, 2013). However, there is an urgent need to refocus limited research dollars and studies toward this community. While 5.3% of all US adults over the age of 50 live with dementia, 7.4% of LGBTQ+ US adults over the age of 50 live with dementia (Alzheimer's Association, 2019; Alzheimer's Association & SAGE, 2018; American Association of Retired Persons, 2014). Generally, LGBTQ+ individuals experience greater health disparities that put them at increased risk for dementia. For example, risk factors for dementia (e.g., depression, obesity, alcohol, and tobacco use, lower rates of preventive screenings, cardiovascular disease, and HIV/AIDS) are more prevalent within the LGBTQ+ population than in the general population (Alzheimer's Association & SAGE, 2018). In seeking dementia care, LGBTQ+ people face greater challenges than the general population because socioeconomic factors undergird whether access to quality care is feasible. A third of LGBTQ+ older adults live at or below 200% of the Federal Poverty Line, rendering dementia-related health services such as respite care, nursing homes, and neuropsychological evaluations less accessible (MAP, 2017).

Older LGBTQ+ adults' experiences of dementia are further nuanced by the diversity within the community. While the population of "older adults" is sometimes defined as broadly as anyone over the age of 50, generational differences are present: a 2016 Gallup poll found that 2.4% of Baby Boomers aged 52–71 identified as LGBTQ+, whereas only 1.4% of Traditionalists[3] aged 72+ identified as LGBTQ+ (Gates, 2017). Racial and ethnic diversity also exist among LGBTQ+ older adults, with 20% of individuals identifying as people of color (Adams, 2016). By 2060, 40% of older LGBTQ+ adults are expected to identify as people of color. Even within the LGBTQ+ community, it is well-documented that gender minority adults experience more health disparities and barriers to health care access than sexual minority adults. Furthermore, gender disparities impact this population. Because women tend to live longer than men, more women are affected by dementia than men, overall; consequently, older lesbians and bisexual women are likely to be disproportionately affected by dementia compared with older gay and bisexual men (Westwood, 2014). Literature documenting dementia trends among LGBTQ+ people is scarce and mixed in results. One study found that older LGBTQ+ individuals in same sex relationships showed less functional impairment and less steep decline in working memory compared to mixed sex relationships, possibly related to protective factors (Correro Ii et al., 2023).

This chapter will explore the current literature and highlight the urgency of directing additional research toward LGBTQ+ older adults. First, the chapter will present extant data demonstrating that LGBTQ+ older adults constitute a vulnerable population with respect to AD/ADRD, with a special emphasis on psychosocial factors that impact both LGBTQ+ individuals and their caregivers. Next, the chapter will describe theoretical constructs that guide research examining the multiplicative, interactive experiences of LGBTQ+ older adults, including racial and ethnic minoritized groups, people living with HIV/AIDS and transgender populations. These constructs include the intersectionality and syndemics frameworks, which work together to capture the experiences of multiple marginalized populations.

CONCERNS AMONG LGBTQ+ ADULTS

Discrimination at the Micro-, Mezzo-, and Macro-Levels

While fear is common among older adults diagnosed with dementia and their caregivers, LGBTQ+ older adults additionally face fear of discrimination on the basis of their sexual orientation, gender identity, and gender expression. This discrimination impacts LGBTQ+ experiences of dementia at all levels of influence: the "micro," the interpersonal or individual level; the "mezzo," the community or organizational level; and the "macro," the state, federal, or societal level governing policies.

At the individual and interpersonal levels, LGBTQ+ older adults' experiences of dementia are characterized by a lack of understanding and empathy from providers, nursing homes, and other dementia-related agencies. In relation to senior housing agencies, which often provide care for individuals with AD/ADRD, older LGBTQ+ adults reported significant anxiety, apprehension, and fear of discrimination and abuse from staff, caregivers, management, and other residents (Stein et al., 2009). These fears are not unfounded: LGBTQ+ older adults have reported barriers to gender expression, especially in care homes (Benbow & Beeston, 2012). Additionally, providers' lack of cultural competence leads to interactions with LGBTQ+ older adults that may discourage them from returning in the future or disclosing important aspects of their identities (Brennan-Ing et al., 2013). Examples of these interactions include providers consistently misgendering a transgender individual or refusing to acknowledge LGBTQ+ individuals' partners.

Stigma associated with LGBTQ+ identities at the individual and interpersonal levels impacts older LGBTQ+ adults in terms of access to care as well as care itself. LGBTQ+

older adults may delay or avoid essential preventive care and neuropsychiatric screenings related to dementia. If an older LGBTQ+ adult does visit their provider, the fear of discrimination may negatively impact diagnosis and receipt of care. In one study, 40% of LGBTQ+ older adults in their sixties and seventies indicated that their health care providers did not know their sexual orientation or identity (SAGE, 2014). While this may seem somewhat inconsequential, this lack of disclosure may translate to further nondisclosure of important medical procedures and history associated with non-heteronormative identities, such as gender-reassignment surgery, hormone therapy, or HIV pre-exposure prophylaxis medication. Equally important, experiences with providers should be humanizing: living with AD/ADRD can be a debilitating experience that leaves many older adults feeling vulnerable. Providers and senior homes can play a crucial role in alleviating the stress that comes with dementia and, therefore, have a responsibility to understand and accommodate the unique stressors experienced by LGBTQ+ older adults living with dementia.

At the organizational and community levels, agency decisions and policies may fail to meet the needs of older LGBTQ+ adults with AD/ADRD. In a study examining 84 providers in the metropolitan Minneapolis-St. Paul Area, 97.6% had no specific services for gay and lesbian older adults, and 94% had no outreach to the LGBTQ+ community (Knochel et al., 2010). Similarly, a survey of Michigan aging services providers demonstrated that LGBTQ+ aging was not a priority for agencies, with little outreach, programming, and planning in place (Hughes et al., 2011). The lack of programming and outreach at the mezzo level likely reflects both a lack of research among LGBTQ+ older adults as well as macro-level policy directives of state and federal governments that exclude this population.

Historically, there is rampant macro-level policy discrimination in housing, hospitals, care centers, and legal rights for LGBTQ+ individuals (Cohen et al., 2008). State policies dictating official gender and name changes, for example, may impact the types of care accessible to transgender older adults living with AD/ADRD. Long-term dementia care centers that only accept individuals who were assigned the sex, "female," at birth may not admit a transgender woman who lives in a state where they cannot legally change their gender identity. Those who do not identify in the gender binary as either man or woman may face additional barriers when searching for gender-neutral options for dementia care. Furthermore, general macro-level policy related to dementia care tends to disproportionately affect LGBTQ+ older adults. For example, Medicare and commercial insurers do not compensate caregivers for the out-of-pocket living expenses associated with dementia care. These expenses fall on caregivers and families, who bear 70% of the total overall cost of an individual living with dementia, estimated at $225,140 per individual, from diagnosis to death (Jutkowitz et al., 2017). Since one-third of LGBTQ+ older adults currently live at or below 200% of the Federal Poverty Line, paying for the basic necessities associated with at-home care without financial support may be unfeasible (MAP, 2017).

These multilevel experiences of discrimination and stigma are not only felt by LGBTQ+ older adults but also by the broader LGBTQ+ community. Instances of discrimination at the individual level that take place throughout the life course compound to form larger narratives of medical mistrust across the entire LGBTQ+ community. Thus, discrimination and fear at the micro level inform community- and population-level interactions between the LGBTQ+ older adult population and health care systems. Furthermore, policy decisions at the mezzo and macro levels impact available treatment options and access to care for LGBTQ+ older adults with dementia, increasing barriers to the receipt of care among this population. This cycle influences the ways in which dementia develops and worsens among LGBTQ+ older adults and contributes to the vulnerability of this community in the face of AD/ADRD and other neurodegenerative diseases.

LGBTQ+ Isolation and Caregiver Stress

Generally, aging with dementia comes with its own set of isolating conditions: people with dementia tend to withdraw from situations that provide social support, exacerbating social isolation (Alzheimer's Association, 2012). Stigma attached to dementia and aging is widespread and has profound effects on how dementia is experienced by individuals (Graham et al., 2003). In many cases, stigma against older adults with dementia impacts the "humanity" of individuals. In place of the various attributes and features that form an individual's identity, "having dementia" becomes their most prominent characteristic (Goffman, 2022). Combined with the negative stigma and fear surrounding dementia, older people diagnosed with dementia are relegated to a "lower status social group" and face social isolation (Katsuno, 2005). In this way, stigma and isolation operate as a feedback loop, potentially worsening the symptoms of older adults with dementia: being diagnosed with dementia catalyzes stigmatizing attitudes that isolate individuals and isolating conditions prevent individuals from accessing social support and resources that may slow the degenerative effects of dementia. Therefore, it is important to consider how social engagement can improve or protect cognitive functioning of individuals with dementia (Vance et al., 2013).

While older adults with dementia may experience isolation, those who identify as LGBTQ+ face additional circumstances that exacerbate this isolation. Stigma and discrimination toward LGBTQ+ individuals manifest during interactions related to their sexuality, family members, and various geographies, such as the "coming out" process and establishing LGBTQ+ domestic partnerships. These socio-geographic interactions result in fewer available social support resources and a lack of family support, which, in turn, translates to fewer available resources for LGBTQ+ older adults with dementia and their caregivers.

As they grow older, LGBTQ+ individuals face several "relational turning points" with their family members because of their sexual orientation (Tyler & Abetz, 2022). If LGBTQ+ individuals choose to "come out" of their closet, or disclose their sexual orientation, they face the possibility of being cut off from their immediate family because of anti-LGBTQ+ views. In losing immediate family, LGBTQ+ individuals may lose the social support systems necessary to facilitate dementia care. Indeed, a vast literature describes the family system as an especially important care resource for older adults experiencing any type of illness (Shanas, 1979). Additionally, social factors greatly affect available family support systems. Immigration status is a key example. While for some LGBTQ+ older adults, extended family members may remain a reliable source of support, children of immigrants may not have the same resources because their extended families live thousands of miles away, speak other languages, and have different cultural vocabularies.

Outside of the family system, safety issues and fear of discrimination drive social isolation among LGBTQ+ adults. Examining the lack of protection afforded to LGBTQ+ adults within the American legal system provides evidence of a culture and society that fails to consider the needs of LGBTQ+ individuals. Although gay marriage was legalized in the

United States at the federal level in 2015, a record-shattering number of anti-LGBTQ+ measures were enacted and introduced at the state level in 2021 (Human Rights Campaign, 2021). State initiatives have continued to emerge in 2022. For example, in March 2022, Florida governor Ron DeSantis signed the "Don't Say Gay" bill, a law that essentially banned all discussion of sexual orientation or gender identity in kindergarten through third grade. Public school systems may no longer afford space to children who may be questioning their sexuality or gender identity to discuss their feelings or, potentially, connect with other children having similar thoughts. The Florida legislation reflects an earlier, long-standing federal policy – "Don't Ask, Don't Tell" – which governed the US military from 1994 to 2011. While that policy replaced a full ban on homosexuals serving in the military prior to 1994, it set a discriminatory standard that LGBTQ+ people should not disclose their sexuality to the military or any other federal organizations.

A socio-legal culture that punishes or discourages discussion of sexual orientation in public systems creates a dangerous environment for LGBTQ+ people who want to be open about their identity or actively engage in relationships within their communities. Alden and Parker (2006) found that macro-level antigay beliefs directly contribute to an increase in incidents of hate crimes. Purposefully not disclosing sexual orientation or openly engaging in meaningful nonheterosexual relationships can be a legitimate and logical tactic to ensure safety among LGBTQ+ individuals. Indeed, a New York City community-level study suggested that greater gay visibility consistently predicts higher levels of antigay hate crimes (Mills, 2021). Both legal statutes preventing disclosure of sexuality as well as anti-LGBTQ hate crimes may contribute to LGBTQ+ individuals' social isolation. While the links between these factors have not been studied extensively, extant research demonstrates that LGBTQ+ older adults face severe isolation as they age. One nationally representative study demonstrated that two-thirds of heterosexual seniors lived with at least one other person, whereas two-thirds of LGBTQ+ seniors lived alone (American Society on Aging & MetLife, 2010). Additionally, LGBTQ+ older adults are more likely to age without a spouse or partner, more likely to live alone, and less likely to have children to support them (MAP, 2010).

In cases where LGBTQ+ older adults with dementia may live with a caregiver, social isolation and discriminatory experiences create stressful caregiver experiences. For spouses and other caregivers of people with dementia, community support and home-based health care services often serve as critical components of dementia care (Newbronner et al., 2013). However, seeking these services and programs as a spouse or caregiver of an LGBTQ+ older adult oftentimes means disclosing the sexual orientation and partnership status of both individuals. Also, due to existing homophobic sentiment, LGBTQ+ individuals may experience anxiety about how to disclose sexuality to service providers who may come into their homes to provide or arrange care (Newman & Price, 2012). This aspect of caregiver stress may be exacerbated by not having immediate or extended family as a support system, as some research has shown that LGBTQ+ adults are less dependent on their families of origin for support, as compared to heterosexual adults (Grossman et al., 2000). One promising study, however, showed that the widely used Savvy Caregiver Program could be tailored and implemented successfully for LGBTQ+ people. The study demonstrated improvements in self-efficacy, caregiver mastery, and increases in social support for caregivers, suggesting that caregivers' feelings of being ill-equipped to navigate the health care system for LGBTQ+ individuals with AD/ADRD can be addressed through tailored programming for this group (Kittle et al., 2022).

Throughout their lifetimes, LGBTQ+ older adults with dementia experience discrimination on the basis of their sexual orientation that is shaped by policy decisions, social interactions, and stigmatizing experiences. Though isolation is not necessarily preferred, it is oftentimes required of LGBTQ+ individuals as a way to preserve their sense of safety from harassment and hate crimes. With few social connections, scant practical resources, and limited caregiver support, LGBTQ+ older adults with dementia may lack crucial means for slowing the progression of their disease. In parallel, LGBTQ+ caregivers – spouses in particular – experience increased caregiving burden because they often lack family support and have difficulties in disclosing their sexuality to health care providers and home health aides. Future studies exploring the different pathways through which stigma and discrimination impact aging among LGBTQ+ individuals will be critical to improving health outcomes and overall well-being in this population.

WORKING TOWARD AN INTERSECTIONAL SYNDEMICS FRAMEWORK

An emerging theme throughout this chapter is how multiple, intersecting experiences of aging and LGBTQ+ identities compound to create challenging circumstances for older LGBTQ+ individuals with dementia. Yet age and sexual identity are two of many identities that impact how dementia is felt and seen. This section introduces an intersectional syndemics framework to more fully capture the experiences of those with various marginalized identities and co-occurring disorders.

Coined by Kimberlé Crenshaw in 1989, "intersectionality" describes the ways in which systems of oppression overlap and create distinct experiences for people holding multiple identity categories. Most importantly, the intersecting experiences of these people are not merely additive but also multiplicative. For example, LGBTQ+ older adults with dementia experience isolation due to the stigma attached to their illness as well as their nonheterosexual identities. In addition to the isolation resulting from discrimination toward both dementia and nonheterosexual identities, caregivers of LGBTQ+ older adults – who are often their partners or spouses – face the challenge of navigating care systems that may not acknowledge or accept a nontraditional marriage. In this way, intersectionality underscores the importance of investigating distinct phenomena (e.g., disproportionate caregiver burden for LGBTQ+ older adults) that emerge at the intersection of multiple marginalized identities.

Syndemics complements the intersectionality framework by acknowledging the macro-level psychosocial forces that contribute to the rise of co-occurring epidemics. These epidemics work in tandem to undermine health in especially vulnerable populations, including LGBTQ+ older adults (Singer & Clair, 2003). Rather than focusing on a single disease, syndemics acknowledges that individuals may experience multiple health issues simultaneously, enabling a holistic understanding of well-being that takes into account the social, psychological and economic conditions impacting individual health. For example, systemic homophobic policies (e.g., state policies dictating official gender and name changes) contribute to the persistent lack of appropriate health and social services for older LGBTQ+ adults. This dearth of services, in turn, contributes to higher rates of dementia and other chronic diseases in this population, such as HIV/AIDS, diabetes, and cardiovascular disease (SAGE, 2013). These co-occurring epidemics have deleterious effects on older LGBTQ+ adults, with some research demonstrating that those living in highly stigmatized environments may experience a life expectancy that is 12 years shorter than non-LGBTQ people (Hatzenbuehler, 2014).

An intersectional syndemics framework operates by identifying the macro-level psychosocial forces that disproportionately impact individuals with multiple marginalized identities, catalyzing co-occurring epidemics that harm their well-being. The next subsections will illustrate this concept by highlighting the dementia-related experiences of 1) LGBTQ+ older adults who are members of racial and ethnic minoritized groups and 2) transgender older adults. These two examples will underscore how systemic forces, rather than individual-level factors or choices, create co-occurring epidemics of HIV/AIDS and mental illness that greatly decrease the quality of life of individuals with these identities.

Racial and Ethnic Minoritized Communities and HIV/AIDS

LGBTQ+ older adults belonging to racial and ethnic minoritized communities, particularly Black and Brown communities, are disproportionately impacted by systemic discrimination. There remains a lack of research about these communities because sufficient funding has not been allocated to understanding their needs. Older LGBTQ+ people of color essentially hold "triple-minority status," with no dedicated source of stable funding to explore the needs of this aggregate population. Instead, researchers must cobble together separate funding streams serving the needs of LGBTQ+ individuals, people of color, and older individuals (Kimmel, 2013). With little research to guide the allocation of federal and local resources, government agencies, in turn, are disincentivized to fund specialized programs that investigate and address health disparities.

The limited evidence available demonstrates that older LGBTQ+ individuals of color are impacted by macro-level discrimination and policy decisions in multiple ways. Black and Brown communities tend to have lower socioeconomic status due to persistent discriminatory practices at the federal level. Throughout American history, governmental policies have excluded these communities purposefully from participating in and benefiting from welfare programs (Stoesz, 2016). Certainly, these policies also affect Black and Brown LGBTQ+ older adults: Black and Latine LGBTQ+ older adults have lower levels of household income, social support, and educational attainment and experience higher levels of stigma than other groups throughout their lifetime (LGBT+ National Aging Research Center, 2017). Since socioeconomic status impacts access to care and is an important social determinant of health, lower socioeconomic status is often associated with higher disease burden and a lack of health care access (Cutler et al., 2008). Indeed, race has a substantial influence on the prevalence of AD/ADRD, with older Black people being twice as likely to have AD than older non-Hispanic White (White) people but significantly less likely to receive a diagnosis (Alzheimer's Association, 2017).

Macro-level forces have also contributed to the rise of the HIV/AIDS epidemic among Black gay and bisexual men. In 2021, US President Joseph R. Biden released a National HIV/AIDS strategic plan that pointed to racism and lack of health care access as major contributors to HIV-related outcomes and disparities (The White House, 2021). The Centers for Disease Control and Prevention reported that an estimated 26% of all new HIV infections in the United States in 2019 were among Black gay and bisexual men (CDC, 2021). Given that HIV/AIDS and mental illness are risk factors for dementia, it is likely that these illnesses may be contributing to an epidemic of dementia as well. As LGBTQ+ individuals living with HIV grow older, approximately 50% of individuals will experience cognitive problems and HIV-associated dementia will occur in approximately 10–15% of all individuals with HIV (Heaton et al., 2010; McArthur & Brew, 2010). To comprehensively address these co-occurring epidemics in these multiple marginalized groups of LGBTQ+ older adults, researchers and policymakers may benefit from utilizing an intersectional syndemics framework that identifies and underscores the systemic change necessary to address the rising HIV and dementia epidemics within LGBTQ+ older individuals of color.

Transgender Populations and Mental Health

Among LGBTQ+ individuals with dementia, transgender people are especially vulnerable to experiencing social isolation and mental illness. Sixty-five percent of transgender adults feel they will have limited access to health care as they age (SAGE, 2014). Transgender adults face unique challenges related to disclosing or hiding their identity when receiving assistance with tasks such as bathing and dressing, yet neither institutional nor home-based transgender-affirming dementia care is widely available. Experiences of discrimination within the transgender community are prevalent, and a National Center for Transgender Equality report (2015) found that 33% of transgender adults reported a negative interaction with a medical provider during the past year. Narratives of discrimination discourage transgender people from seeking out necessary dementia care, as evidenced by 23% of transgender people reporting that they did not see a doctor when they needed medical care in the prior year (2015).

Discrimination also contributes to social isolation, increasing the risk of co-occurring epidemics of mental illness and depression among transgender older adults. As a subset of the general LGBTQ+ population, transgender individuals have been found to have higher odds of depression symptoms and attempted suicides than non-transgender LGBTQ+ individuals in the United States (Su et al., 2016). National data also show transgender adults report greater subjective cognitive decline, with racial and ethnic minoritized, transgender adults having the highest rates of subjective cognitive decline prevalence compared to both racial and ethnic minoritized and White, cisgender adults (Cicero et al., 2023). In parallel, a recent cohort study in Ireland showed that 78% of transgender people have considered suicide (Transgender Equality Network Ireland, 2013). Research is needed to explore the co-occurrence of mental illness and dementia within older transgender individuals, with particular emphasis on the impacts of cultural norms as well as macro-, mezzo-, and micro-level discrimination.

CONCLUSION

This chapter explores how individuals situated at the intersection of LGBTQ+ identity and older age experience dementia in the United States. While numerous psychosocial factors influence dementia outcomes, discrimination at the individual, community, and federal levels contributes to social isolation and reduces access to dementia care. At the same time, there is significant diversity among older LGBTQ+ adults. An intersectional syndemics framework may be an effective tool to guide future research that acknowledges and explores the impact of macro-level psychosocial factors on people with interlocking identities and their experiences of co-occurring disorders. Such a framework could be indispensable to the development of an evidence base from which *tailored* interventions may be designed that more fully capture and address the complex consequences of marginalization among LGBTQ+ older adults. Prioritizing this work with dedicated funding streams will allow for better identification of health disparities and the implementation of interventions that increase older LGBTQ+ adults' longevity and quality of life.

Discussion Questions

1. How are experiences of social isolation similar and different for the general older adult population with dementia and the LGBTQ+ older adult population with dementia?

2. What are some other examples of intersecting identities that may impact dementia care for older LGBTQ+ adults? What macro-level psychosocial factors contribute to this impact?

3. This chapter focuses on policy and psychosocial factors that may contribute to discriminatory experiences for older LGBTQ+ adults with dementia. What are some other factors that may contribute to these experiences?

NOTES

1. *LGBTQ+* is an acronym for lesbian, gay, bisexual, transgender, queer, and others. The "+" represents all other sexual minority identities. This term is ever changing and is synonymous with LGB+, GLBT, and LGB*.

2. *Baby Boomers* refers to the generation of people born in the years following World War II, when there was a temporary increase in birth rates.

3. Traditionalists preceded the Baby Boomer generation and are currently in their mid-to-late 70s or older.

REFERENCES

Adams, M. (2016). An intersectional approach to services and care for LGBT elders. *Generations: Journal of the American Society on Aging, 40*(2), 94–100. https://www.ingentaconnect.com/content/asag/gen/2016/00000040/00000002/art00020

Alden, H. L., & Parker, K. F. (2006). Gender role ideology, homophobia and hate crime: Linking attitudes to macro-level anti-gay and lesbian hate crimes. *Deviant Behavior, 26*(4), 321–343. https://doi.org/10.1080/01639620931614

Alzheimer's Association. (2012). (rep.). People with Alzheimer's disease and other dementias who live alone: In 2012 Alzheimer's disease facts and figures. *Alzheimer's Association.* Retrieved April 1, 2022, from https://www.alz.org/downloads/facts_figures_2012.pdf

Alzheimer's Association. (2017). (rep.). *2017 Alzheimer's Disease Facts and Figures.* Retrieved from https://www.alz.org/documents_custom/2017-facts-and-figures.pdf

Alzheimer's Association. (2019). (rep.). *2019 Alzheimer's Disease Facts and Figures.* Retrieved April 3, 2022, from https://www.alz.org/media/Documents/alzheimers-facts-and-figures-2019-r.pdf

Alzheimer's Association, & SAGE. (2018). (rep.). *LGBT Older Adults and Dementia.* Retrieved March 25, 2022, from https://www.alz.org/media/Documents/lgbt_older_adults_dementia_infographic.pdf

American Association of Retired Persons. (2014). (rep.). *Getting to Know Americans Age 50+.* AARP. Retrieved April 1, 2022, from https://www.aarp.org/content/dam/aarp/research/surveys_statistics/general/2014/getting-to-know-americans-age-50-plus-demographics.doi.10.26419%252Fres.00091.001.pdf

American Society on Aging, & MetLife. (2010). (rep.). *Still Out, Still Aging: The MetLife Study of Lesbian, Gay, Bisexual, and Transgender Baby Boomers.* Retrieved April 1, 2022, from https://www.asaging.org/sites/default/files/files/mmi-still-out-still-aging.pdf

Benbow, S. M., & Beeston, D. (2012). Sexuality, aging, and dementia. *International Psychogeriatrics, 24*(7), 1026–1033. https://doi.org/10.1017/s1041610212000257

Brennan-Ing, M., Seidel, L., Larson, B., & Karpiak, S. E. (2013). Social care networks and older LGBT adults: Challenges for the future. *Journal of Homosexuality, 61*(1), 21–52. https://doi.org/10.1080/00918369.2013.835235

Centers for Disease Control and Prevention. (2021). (rep.) Estimated HIV incidence and prevalence in the United States, 2015–2019. HIV surveillance supplemental report. Retrieved March 29, 2022 from http://www.cdc.gov/hiv/library/reports/hiv-surveillance.html

Choi, S. K., & Meyer, I. H. (2016). *LGBT Aging: A Review of Research Findings, Needs, and Policy Implications.* The Williams Institute.

Cicero, E. C., Lett, E., Flatt, J. D., Benson, G. P., & Epps, F. (2023). Transgender adults from minoritized ethnoracial groups in the U.S. report greater subjective cognitive decline. *The Journals of Gerontology. Series B, Psychological Sciences and Social Sciences*, gbad012. Advance online publication. https://doi.org/10.1093/geronb/gbad012

Cohen, H. L., Curry, L. C., Jenkins, D., Walker, C. A., & Hogstel, M. O. (2008). Older lesbians and gay men: Long-term care issues. *Annals of Long-Term Care, 16*(2), 33–38. https://www.hmpgloballearningnetwork.com/site/altc/article/8315

Correro, A. N.,II Gauthreaux, K., Perales-Puchalt, J., Chen, Y. C., Chan, K. C. G., Kukull, W. A., & Flatt, J. D. (2023). Cognitive aging with Dementia, Mild cognitive impairment, or no impairment: A comparison of same- and mixed-sex couples. *Journal of Alzheimer's Disease: JAD, 92*(1), 109–128. https://doi.org/10.3233/JAD-220309

Cutler, D., Lleras-Muney, A., & Vogl, T. (2008). *Socioeconomic status and Health: Dimensions and mechanisms.* National Bureau of Economic Research Working Paper No.14333. Available at. https://doi.org/10.3386/w14333.

Gates, G. J. (2017, January 11). In U.S., more adults identifying as LGBT. *Gallup.com.* Gallup. Retrieved April 2, 2022, from http://www.gallup.com/poll/201731/lgbt-identification-rises.aspx

Goffman, E. (2022). *Stigma: Notes on the management of spoiled identity.* Penguin Books.

Graham, N., Lindesay, J., Katona, C., Bertolote, J. M., Camus, V., Copeland, J. R., de Mendonça Lima, C. A., Gaillard, M., Gély Nargeot, M. C., Gray, J., Jacobsson, L., Kingma, M., Kühne, N., O'Loughlin, A., Rutz, W., Saraceno, B., Taintor, Z., & Wancata, J. (2003). Reducing stigma and discrimination against older people with mental disorders: A technical consensus statement. *International Journal of Geriatric Psychiatry, 18*(8), 670–678. https://doi.org/10.1002/gps.876

Grossman, A. H., D'Augelli, A. R., & Hershberger, S. L. (2000). Social support networks of lesbian, gay, and bisexual adults 60 years of age and older. *The Journals of Gerontology Series B: Psychological Sciences and Social Sciences, 55*(3), 171–179. https://doi.org/10.1093/geronb/55.3.p171

Hatzenbuehler, M. L. (2014). Structural stigma and the health of Lesbian, gay, and bisexual populations. *Current Directions in Psychological Science, 23*(2), 127–132. https://doi.org/10.1177/0963721414523775

Heaton, R. K., Clifford, D. B., Franklin, D. R., Jr, Woods, S. P., Ake, C., Vaida, F., Ellis, R. J., Letendre, S. L., Marcotte, T. D., Atkinson, J. H., Rivera-Mindt, M., Vigil, O. R., Taylor, M. J., Collier, A. C., Marra, C. M., Gelman, B. B., McArthur, J. C., Morgello, S., Simpson, D. M., & McCutchan, J. A., & CHARTER Group. (2010). HIV-associated neurocognitive disorders persist in the era of potent antiretroviral therapy: CHARTER study. *Neurology, 75*(23), 2087–2096. https://doi.org/10.1212/WNL.0b013e318200d727

Hughes, A. K., Harold, R. D., & Boyer, J. M. (2011). Awareness of LGBT aging issues among aging services network providers. *Journal of Gerontological Social Work, 54*(7), 659–677. https://doi.org/10.1080/01634372.2011.585392

Human Rights Campaign. (2021, May 7). 2021 officially becomes worst year in recent history for LGBTQ state legislative attacks as unprecedented number of states enact record-shattering number of Anti-LGBTQ measures into law. *Human Rights Campaign.* Retrieved April 1, 2022, from https://www.hrc.org/press-releases/2021-officially-becomes-worst-year-in-recent-history-for-lgbtq-state-legislative-attacks-as-unprecedented-number-of-states-enact-record-shattering-number-of-anti-lgbtq-measures-into-law

Jones, J. M. (2022, February 18). LGBT identification in U.S. ticks up to 7.1%. *Gallup.com. from* https://news.gallup.com/poll/389792/lgbt-identification-ticks-up.aspx

Jutkowitz, E., Kane, R. L., Gaugler, J. E., MacLehose, R. F., Dowd, B., & Kuntz, K. M. (2017). Societal and family lifetime cost of dementia: Implications for policy. *Journal of the American Geriatrics Society, 65*(10), 2169–2175. https://doi.org/10.1111/jgs.15043

Katsuno, T. (2005). Dementia from the inside: How people with early-stage dementia evaluate their quality of life. *Ageing and Society, 25*(2), 197–214. https://doi.org/10.1017/s0144686×0400279x

Kimmel, D. (2013). Lesbian, gay, bisexual, and transgender aging concerns. *Clinical Gerontologist, 37*(1), 49–63. https://doi.org/10.1080/07317115.2014.847310

Kittle, K. R., Lee, R., Pollock, K., Song, Y., Wharton, W., Anderson, J. G., Dowling, N. M., & Flatt, J. D. (2022). Feasibility of the savvy caregiver program for LGBTQ+ caregivers of people living with Alzheimer's disease and related Dementias. *International Journal of Environmental Research and Public Health, 19*(22), 15102. https://doi.org/10.3390/ijerph192215102

Knochel, K. A., Quam, J. K., & Croghan, C. F. (2010). Are old lesbian and gay people well served? *Journal of Applied Gerontology, 30*(3), 370–389. https://doi.org/10.1177/0733464810369809

LGBT+ National Aging Research Center. (2017). *Aging with Pride: National Health, Aging, and Sexuality/ Gender Study.* The Goldsen Institute. Retrieved April 1, 2022, from http://age-pride.org

McArthur, J. C., & Brew, B. J. (2010). HIV-associated neurocognitive disorders: Is there a hidden epidemic? *AIDS (London, England), 24*(9), 1367–1370. https://doi.org/10.1097/QAD.0b013e3283391d56

McNeil, J., Bailey, L., Ellis, S. J., & Regan, M. (2013). (rep.). *Speaking from the Margins: Trans Mental Health and Wellbeing in Ireland.* Retrieved March 22, 2022, from https://pure.hud.ac.uk/en/publications/ speaking-from-the-margins-trans-mental-health-and-wellbeing-in-ir

Mills, C. E. (2021). Gay visibility and disorganized and strained communities: A community-level analysis of anti-gay hate crime in New York City. *Journal of interpersonal violence, 36*(17-18), 8070–8091. https://doi. org/10.1177/0886260519848784

Movement Advancement Project, & SAGE. (2010). (rep.). *Improving the Lives of hLGBT Older Adults.* Retrieved March 25, 2022, from https://www.lgbtmap.org/file/improving-the-lives-of-lgbt-older-adults.pdf

Movement Advancement Project, & SAGE. (2017). (rep.). *Understanding Issues Facing LGBT Older Adults.* Movement Advancement Project (MAP). Retrieved March 27, 2022, from https://www.lgbtmap.org/file/ understanding-issues-facing-lgbt-older-adults.pdf

National Center for Transgender Equality (NCTE). (2015). *The Report of the 2015 U.S. Transgender Survey.* Retrieved April 1, 2022, from https://transequality.org/sites/default/files/docs/usts/USTS-Full-Report-Dec17.pdf

Newbronner, L., Chamberlain, R., Borthwick, R., Baxter, M., & Glendinning, C. (2013). A road less rocky: Supporting carers of people with dementia. *Research Report.* Carers Trust

Newman, R., & Price, E. (2012). Meeting the needs of LGBT people affected by dementia: The story of the LGBT dementia support group. In R. Ward, I. Rivers, & M. Sutherland (Eds.), *Lesbian, gay, bisexual and transgender ageing: Biographical approaches for inclusive care and support* (pp. 183–195). Jessica Kingsley Publishers.

The White House. (2021). *National HIV/AIDS Strategy for the United States 2022–2025.*

SAGE. (2013). (rep.). *Health Equity and LGBTQ Elders of Color: Recommendations for Policy and Practice.* Retrieved March 28, 2022, from https://www.sageusa.org/wp-content/uploads/2018/06/2013-sage-health-equity-and-lgbt-elders-recommendations-for-policy-and-practice-2.pdf

SAGE. (2014). (rep.). *Out & Visible The Experiences and Attitudes of Lesbian, Gay, Bisexual and Transgender Older Adults, Ages 45–75.* Retrieved April 1, 2022, from https://www.sageusa.org/wp-content/uploads/2018/05/ sageusa-out-visible-lgbt-market-research-full-report.pdf

Shanas, E. (1979). The family as a social support system in old age. *The Gerontologist, 19*(2), 169–174. https:// doi.org/10.1093/geront/19.2.169

Singer, M., & Clair, S. (2003). Syndemics and public health: Reconceptualizing disease in bio-social context. *Medical Anthropology Quarterly, 17*(4), 423–441. https://doi.org/10.1525/maq.2003.17.4.423

Stein, G. L., Beckerman, N. L., & Sherman, P. A. (2009). Lesbian and gay elders and long-term care: Identifying the unique psychosocial perspectives and challenges. *Journal of Gerontological Social Work, 53*(5), 421–435. https://doi.org/10.1080/01634372.2010.496478

Stoesz, D. (2016). The excluded: An estimate of the consequences of denying Social Security to agricultural and domestic workers (CSD Working Paper No. 16–17). Washington University, Center for Social Development.

Su, D., Irwin, J. A., Fisher, C., Ramos, A., Kelley, M., Mendoza, D. A., & Coleman, J. D. (2016). Mental health disparities within the LGBT population: A comparison between transgender and nontransgender individuals. *Transgender Health, 1*(1), 12–20. https://doi.org/10.1089/trgh.2015.0001

Transgender Equality Network Ireland. (2013). (rep.). *STAD: Stop Transphobia and Discrimination Report.* Transgender Equality Network Ireland. Retrieved from https://teni.ie/wp-content/uploads/2019/07/STAD-2013.pdf.

Tyler, T. R., & Abetz, J. S. (2022). Relational turning points in the parent and LGBTQ child coming out process. *Journal of Family Studies, 28*(3), 858–878. https://doi.org/10.1080/13229400.2020.1761863

Urban Institute. (2022). The US population is aging. Retrieved April 1, 2022, from https://www.urban.org/policy-centers/cross-center-initiatives/program-retirement-policy/projects/data-warehouse/what-future-holds/us-population-aging

Vance, D. E., Fazeli, P. L., Moneyham, L., Keltner, N. L., & Raper, J. L. (2013). Assessing and treating forgetfulness and cognitive problems in adults with HIV. *The Journal of the Association of Nurses in AIDS Care: JANAC*, *24*(1 Suppl), S40–S60. https://doi.org/10.1016/j.jana.2012.03.006

Westwood, S. (2014). Dementia, women and sexuality: How the intersection of ageing, gender and sexuality magnify dementia concerns among lesbian and bisexual women. *Dementia*, *15*(6), 1494–1514. https://doi.org/10.1177/1471301214564446

CHAPTER

COMMUNITY AND PATIENT ENGAGEMENT OF OLDER ADULTS IN AGING AND ALZHEIMER'S DISEASE AND ALZHEIMER'S DISEASE-RELATED DEMENTIAS RESEARCH

CHAU TRINH-SHEVRIN, RACHEL SACKS, JEANNETTE MICHELE BEASLEY,
NISHA GODBOLE, AISHA T. LANGFORD, SCOTT E. SHERMAN,
JOSHUA CHODOSH

LEARNING OBJECTIVES

By the end of this chapter, readers will be able to:

- Understand challenges in engaging older populations in clinical trials research, including studies of cognitive impairment and Alzheimer's disease and Alzheimer's disease-related dementias (AD/ADRD) among communities of racial and ethnic minoritized and low-income adults over 65.

- Apply participatory and health communication frameworks in community and patient engagement relevant to older populations, particularly those identifying as being from minoritized and low-income groups.
- Identify electronic health record (EHR)- and community health worker (CHW)-based strategies to improve engagement, recruitment, and retention of older adults in clinical trials and community-based studies.

INTRODUCTION

As discussed in Chapter 1, demographic shifts in the United States (US) population are transforming the profile of older communities in the US (Ortman et al., 2014). To keep pace with these changing demographics and develop a better understanding of population health needs, research focused on older persons is urgently needed. Significant knowledge gaps exist across the health spectrum spanning prevention, diagnosis, early detection, management, and treatment of chronic and co-occurring conditions, including Alzheimer's disease and Alzheimer's disease-related dementias (AD/ADRD), among racial and ethnic minoritized and low-income adults over 65 years old due to barriers in recruiting this diverse population and age category into behavioral and biomedical research (Ortman et al., 2014; Rich et al., 2016). Developing and implementing novel engagement, recruitment, and retention strategies relevant to a broad spectrum of the older adult population is particularly salient to addressing these gaps (Sood & Stahl, 2011).

This chapter will describe ways in which researchers, public health professionals, clinicians, and communities can work together toward increasing participation of those who are 65 years and older from racial and ethnic minoritized and low-income populations in clinical trials. First, we will discuss challenges to engagement and recruitment of these communities. Second, we will introduce participatory research principles. Third, we will describe a conceptual model and approach for engagement, recruitment, and retention of older adult communities in aging and AD/ADRD research. Fourth, we will discuss specific recruitment methods that harness both technological and human resources and best practices to enhance recruitment and retention of older racial and ethnic minoritized and low-income adults in clinical research.

UNDERSTANDING CHALLENGES

Comorbidity among older individuals ages 65 and older represents a critical area of study for aging and AD/ADRD researchers. Aging demographics drive chronic comorbid conditions, frailty, and the need for better evidence on prevention, diagnosis, early detection, management, and treatment of chronic and co-occurring conditions. The accumulation of chronic comorbid conditions is more strongly associated with age than with any other human characteristic (Murray et al., 2013), resulting in functional disabilities and loss of independence (Stenholm et al., 2015). Many clinical, psychosocial, and physiological risk factors are modifiable, yet tremendous knowledge gaps persist related to their role and impact on outcomes.

Within the few funded studies that focus on these issues, researchers often struggle to achieve recruitment and retention goals. Research participation has steadily declined over the past 30 years overall (Galea & Tracy, 2007). Despite tremendous population growth, older persons, particularly of racial and ethnic minoritized groups, participate in research studies at levels far below their population prevalence (A. L. Gilmore-Bykovskyi et al., 2019; Konkel, 2015; Ta Park et al., 2021). For example, non-Hispanic Black (Black) and (Hispanic) Latine people comprise 30% of the US population; however, they only make up 6% of all participants in government-funded clinical trials (Konkel, 2015). Older participants have been underrepresented in cardiovascular and cancer trials (Langford et al., 2014; Michelet et al., 2014; Rich et al., 2016) and, typically, clinical trials for these and other conditions, including AD/ADRD, exclude older patients with complex comorbidities, significant physical or cognitive disabilities, frailty, or residence in a nursing home or assisted living facility (Mangoni et al., 2013; Michelet et al., 2014; Shipman et al., 2008). Yet, at the same time, cancer and other chronic conditions are more often diagnosed in individuals aged 65 years or older, rendering advanced age a key risk factor, which requires older adults be included in clinical trials to better understand these conditions (Langford et al., 2014). Comorbidities are a common reason for clinical trial ineligibility but an important consideration when designing protocols, due to their impact on the condition of interest (Kotler & Zaltman, 1971; Langford et al., 2014). However, expanding clinical trials to include older participants with comorbidities is critical because those with multiple chronic conditions may receive less benefit from guideline-concordant care while simultaneously experiencing more adverse effects from treatment. Furthermore, evidence of "what works" is less generalizable for those with multiple chronic conditions and/or from racial and ethnic minoritized populations. The full spectrum of older people in clinical research is needed to develop better guidelines and reduce the disproportionate burden of health disparities among low-income and racial and ethnic minoritized communities (Ashing-Giwa & Rosales, 2012; James et al., 2017; McDougall et al., 2015).

Older-age participants face sensitivities that differ from younger-age participants in recruitment and retention in human subjects' research, highlighting a need for logistical and administrative strategies to address these issues (Anderson et al., 2000; Mody et al., 2008). Examples include concerns about mobility, cognitive impairment, the need for a care partner to accompany a participant, and capacity to consent limiting access to research opportunities. Mobility issues raise needs for transportation and may unfairly exclude otherwise eligible research subject candidates (Witham & McMurdo, 2007). Incentives and enablers may be needed to compensate the time and effort of care partners and able-bodied companions accompanying frail or physically challenged participants to study visits. Offering flexible appointments and virtual visits (i.e., in order to account for digital access issues) may also expand the population who may be able to participate (Langford & Bateman-House, 2020). Meanwhile, candidates with mild to moderate cognitive impairment are often excluded due to concerns of decisional capacity (i.e., consent); however, many of these individuals have maintained capacity to consent and may benefit from research participation. Functional disabilities, including communication disabilities (e.g., hearing and vision loss), require strategies to avoid indiscriminate exclusion, tailoring consent language and requirements, adequate time allotment for intervention delivery, and flexible survey administration and data collection methods (Cohen et al., 2017; Djuric et al., 2012; Normansell et al., 2016).

Despite the health-related and economic barriers unique to older adults, research has shown that people aged 70 years and older have more favorable views of research participation and a greater willingness to participate than younger counterparts (Comis et al., 2003; Peterson et al., 2004). Moreover, this willingness is independent of trial outcomes (Schron et al., 1997; Yuval et al., 2001). As patients, those who are older have more frequent interactions with the health care system than those who are younger, providing more opportunities to engage in research. Yet few older persons who might benefit from being in a clinical trial are proactive in seeking information, requiring facilitated efforts to engage and navigate older-age individuals toward relevant studies (Townsley et al., 2006). This is particularly true for people from racial and ethnic minoritized and immigrant older communities, who may have low health literacy and limited English proficiency (Becerra et al., 2017; Kamimura et al., 2013). The lack of understanding and trust among potential participants of what clinical trials are and how research may benefit them and their communities is intensified and exacerbated by ageist biases and stereotypes that remain widespread among providers, researchers, and policymakers (Petrovsky et al., 2022). While toolkits have been developed to support recruitment efforts and share information about clinical trial participation (National Institute on Aging, 2015), these resources focus on addressing patient-, provider-, and community-level misconceptions about the value of research rather than addressing ageist biases among the research community (Ford et al., 2008; Hanson et al., 2010). There remains not only a persistent need for effective methods to build trust among potential participants and trial administrators but also for resources to engage both providers and the population at large in thinking about older adults. This is particularly true for people from racial and ethnic minoritized and low-income communities that have been subjected to historical systemic abuse by public health authorities and scientific research teams (e.g., the Tuskegee syphilis study) (Centers for Disease Control and Prevention, 2022).

APPLYING COMMUNITY-ENGAGED RESEARCH PRINCIPLES

Community-engaged research principles may provide important foundational guidance for building this trust and supporting the recruitment and retention of participants in AD/ADRD research overall (Table 5.1). Community-based participatory research (CBPR) is a form of community-engaged research that actively involves community members throughout the research process. Increasingly, CBPR is viewed as a framework for facilitating collaboration between community members and academic researchers (D'Alonzo, 2010; Meade et al., 2011; Trinh-Shevrin et al., 2007; Wallerstein & Duran, 2010).

The establishment of the federal Patient Centered Outcomes Research Institute (PCORI) provided an important mechanism for increasing community-engaged research (Patient Protection and Affordable Care Act, 2010), by focusing attention on how and why researchers should prioritize the engagement of individual patients, their care partners, and their families in research (Hasnain-Wynia & Beal, 2014). PCORI has helped to expand the definition of those involved in and impacted by research to include providers and payers, along with patients, patient advocacy groups, families, and other care partners. PCORI has also been instrumental in promoting patient engagement strategies such as reaching out to

TABLE 5.1 Guiding Principles and Benefits of CBPR

Guiding CBPR Principles	Benefits of CBPR
• Promotes active community and multisector collaboration and participation at every stage of research, balancing the power dynamics between academic and community partners • Facilitates co-learning and understanding of barriers to trust and engagement in research and an appreciation of the local wisdom of communities in informing research design and solutions • Ensures research/interventions are community-driven and addresses health priorities while accounting for social determinants of health • Disseminates results in useful ways for community members beyond peer review publications to encompass policy briefs and recommendations in ways that are accessible to lay audiences • Ensures research and intervention strategies are culturally and linguistically appropriate • Defines community as a unit of identity, ensuring that the research, solutions, and findings are localized within the community context	• Fosters trusting relationships between researchers and communities through an understanding and appreciation of contextual factors that inhibit research engagement and a paradigm focused on advancing equitable partnerships • Promotes increased relevance of research questions and goals that are informed by lived experiences of community members • Increases quantity and quality of collected data as community partners are engaged in strengthening outreach, recruitment and retention strategies, and relevance of survey measures • Enhances use and relevance of collected data that can be used by community members and organizations and has direct tangible meaning • Promotes dissemination of findings through multiple channels (publications, infographics, conferences, town halls, mainstream and ethnic media) • Facilitates infrastructure building and sustainability as it builds local community capacity to engage in research and is informed by community members and other involved actors

Source: Adapted from Israel et al. 1998.

individuals having a lived experience of a particular illness and to those care partners/ family members involved in their care.

Yet many researchers continue to struggle with how best to engage a wide and diverse group that ensures research is patient-centered, methodologically rigorous in its approach, and generalizable to different populations and settings. Strategies to improve community and multisectoral engagement include the development of patient advisory councils and community advisory boards to contribute to identifying priorities, study design, implementation, evaluation, and dissemination (Bougrab et al., 2019). Given CBPR's emphasis on involving patients, care partners, and family members in the research process, integrating core CBPR principles into study designs can assist researchers in developing more effective and efficient patient-centered research.

A CONCEPTUAL MODEL AND APPROACH FOR CLINICAL TRIAL PARTICIPATION

As CBPR methods are applied to aging and AD/ADRD research, a novel conceptual model may guide the development of tools and strategies to enhance recruitment and retention of older adults in the context of patient–provider encounters. Adults aged 65 and older are more likely to seek health care services due to higher likelihood of illness and need for chronic disease management. Opportunities to engage these older patients, including those from racial and ethnic minoritized communities, have yet to be optimized for clinical trials recruitment. Figure 5.1 presents a conceptual model guided by the work of Aisha T. Langford, PhD, to improve clinical trial participation in the context of vaccine and other clinical trial studies. Additionally, *Assume, Seek, Know* (ASK) is an approach to enhance equity, inclusion, and efficiency built on three underlying principles: researchers should 1) *assume* that all patients will want to know their options; 2) *seek* the counsel of those involved in research, such as patients and community members; and 3) *know* their numbers (i.e., potentially eligible patients, invitations sent via different channels, response rates, interested but not eligible patients, declines by eligible patients, and enrolled patients) (Langford, 2020).

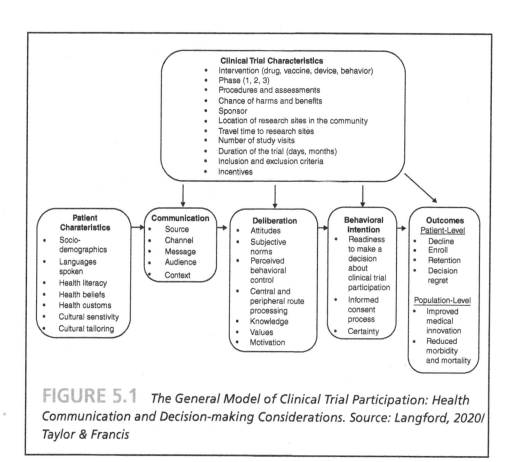

FIGURE 5.1 *The General Model of Clinical Trial Participation: Health Communication and Decision-making Considerations. Source: Langford, 2020/ Taylor & Francis*

The General Model of Clinical Trial Participation presents a framework for considering the relationship among clinical communication, participation, and decision-making that can inform tools and strategies to support the successful recruitment and engagement of older adults in clinical research. Historically, patients were made aware of clinical trials through conversations with a health care provider, especially for health conditions where multiple visits with subspecialists might occur (Ford et al., 2008). In these situations, shared decision-making with clinical providers may help patients decide whether a clinical trial is right for them. More recently, direct-to-consumer invitations (e.g., patient portals, letters, emails, phone calls), national registries (e.g., Research Match), public databases (e.g., ClinicalTrials.gov), and marketing techniques (e.g., paid advertisements on social media) have emerged as other ways patients become aware of clinical trial opportunities.

Notably, finding and understanding information about clinical trials is impacted by personal health literacy, defined by the Centers for Disease Control and Prevention (CDC) within Healthy People 2030 as "the degree to which individuals have the ability to find, understand, and use information and services to inform health-related decisions and actions for themselves and others" (CDC, 2020). Health literacy can also be impacted by language barriers and the need for racially and ethnically concordant researchers who are bilingual (Gilmore-Bykovskyi et al., 2019; Lim et al., 2020; Ta Park et al., 2021; Portacolone et al., 2020).

Once patients are aware of clinical trial opportunities, their intention or willingness to participate is influenced by their preferences for treatment, attitudes about clinical trials, subjective norms, and perceived behavioral control (Steinman et al., 2015). Assuming that a clinical trial is available, intention should lead to key outcomes. As illustrated in Figure 5.1, patient-level outcomes include enrollment, decision quality, retention, decision regret, and population-level outcomes focused on addressing gaps in clinical trial participation and assessing the impact of reduction in related disparities. Additional factors may also impact recruitment and retention, including ageism among providers and researchers and a historical lack of federal guidelines and policies governing inclusion of older people in clinical trials, which has led to the exclusion of many groups of older people, such as those with comorbidities or extremely advanced age (Petrovsky et al., 2022). Other issues may include clinical trial characteristics that preclude participation by some older people (e.g., time burden, tasks required) (Eborall et al., 2011), quality of the informed consent process (Ofstedal & Weir, 2011), and incentives.

DEVELOPING HEALTH MESSAGING AND COMMUNICATIONS

To facilitate implementation of the conceptual model, tailored and appropriate health messaging and communications strategies are critical. Table 5.2 summarizes aspects of health communications and messaging that are essential to supporting successful engagement, recruitment, and retention of racial and ethnic minoritized older adults in clinical research trials.

Health messaging should utilize a common vocabulary and language to describe research that is accessible to laypersons – and racial and ethnic minoritized communities in particular. The careful selection of words, languages, and semantics will be critical to the success of any recruitment and engagement efforts (Ajrouch et al., 2020) to ensure that potential participants may easily understand the research process and goals (Portacolone et al., 2020). Researchers must break down information patiently, address any participant

TABLE 5.2 **Key Considerations in Developing Health Messaging and Communications**

Strategy	Components
Develop clear, appropriate language/messaging	• Carefully select words/languages and semantics • Distill information patiently, clarify participant confusion, be explicit and transparent about the research process • Construct simple explanatory statements to help participants understand the research process and goals
Choose appropriate messengers and communication channels	• Engage researchers who speak the languages of the communities of focus • Employ telephone calls and personal mail rather than email or text messaging reminders • Use social media platforms preferred by each cultural group the study seeks to engage • Develop tailored messaging for caregivers • Employ an in-person recruitment approach that includes the potential participant as well as a trusted family member or close friend with the recruiter
Focus recruitment messaging and communications on communities of interest	• Conduct outreach and engagement at culturally specific or familiar community spaces such as grocery stores, festivals, cultural centers, spiritual centers • Find community-based partners and liaisons who can be involved with study planning and connect with members of underrepresented populations

Source: Godbole, N., et al., 2022 / Oxford University press.

confusion, and be explicit and transparent about the research process (Forsat et al., 2020; Mitchell et al., 2020; Portacolone et al., 2020), while simultaneously demonstrating empathy and building trust and rapport with participants (A. Gilmore-Bykovskyi et al., 2021; Portacolone et al., 2020). Educational statements about the research topic and how participation will help members of their own communities have been shown to be effective messaging strategies (Forsat et al., 2020; A. Gilmore-Bykovskyi et al., 2021; Portacolone et al., 2020). Social marketing – the application of principles drawn from the commercial sector to influence an audience of interest – has been used in recent years to design messaging and communications that encourage and engage communities in beneficial behavioral change to promote health and well-being (Kotler & Zaltman, 1971; Withall et al., 2012). Social marketing principles are especially well-suited for translating complex educational messages and behavior change techniques into ideas and products that will be received and acted upon by a segment of the population (Tanjasiri et al., 2015). These principles may help foster awareness and education on a range of aging, AD/ADRD, and clinical trial opportunities among individual participants and care partners.

While including racially- and ethnically-concordant researchers and recruiters is fundamental to increasing the likelihood that messaging is tailored appropriately and well-received by the communities of focus, at an even more basic level, engaging researchers who show empathy, work to build trust, and speak the language of the community of interest is critical to increasing participation (A. Gilmore-Bykovskyi et al., 2021; Lim et al., 2020; Portacolone et al., 2020; Ta Park et al., 2021). One study found that clinical research coordinators ranked the importance of language concordance higher than gender, age, and race concordance in facilitating the successful implementation of research (Scott et al., 2019).

DESIGNING RECRUITMENT STRATEGIES AND MAXIMIZING RETENTION

To effectively recruit older-age participants from racial and ethnic minoritized and low-income populations, a dual approach is needed that pairs the power of technology with culturally-tailored community-based outreach and support. These same strategies may also contribute to broader approaches to maximize the retention of older-age participants in clinical research.

Electronic Health Record (EHR)-based Strategies

Across the US, most large and small provider practices use electronic health record (EHR) systems to monitor and manage patient encounters and outcomes. These systems can serve as excellent instruments for identifying patients for inclusion in clinical studies because they allow for identification of potential participants based on different data elements that may be considered individually or in combination as study participation criteria. While researchers typically rely on ambulatory diagnostic codes [i.e., international classification of diseases (ICD-10) codes] as the starting point for patient identification, EHRs also allow for stratification by demographic characteristics that are captured consistently, such as age, male and female gender, and some racial and ethnic characteristics (Deane et al., 2020; Forsat et al., 2020). In principle (i.e., if these data are complete), this search facility allows researchers to search for specific groups within the entire patient population of a health system as they conduct initial engagement and recruitment activities. In practice, race/ethnicity categories have been inconsistently collected in EHR and other health data systems (Polubriaginof et al., 2019). Innovative practices, for example, surname analysis or preferred language spoken, can help to improve sampling strategies of understudied or underrepresented communities (Elliott et al., 2009). For example, for a study of diabetes among older adult patients from racial and ethnic minoritized populations, demographic criteria may include patients who are over age 65, belong to a racial or ethnic group other than non-Hispanic White, speak certain languages common among the ethnic groups of interest and other such elements tracked in the EHR. These demographic criteria can be applied in tandem with an algorithm to identify patients with diabetes, which may operationalize such elements as ambulatory ICD-10 codes, pharmacy data, and laboratory tests (Beasley et al., 2021). These selection criteria and search strategies should be developed by collaborative, interdisciplinary teams that include expertise from aging, AD/ADRD, community engagement, health disparities, minority health, informatics, and health communications.

EHRs can also serve as useful tools to facilitate direct contact between researchers and patients. If a health system's institutional review board (IRB) has allowed for an "opt-out" process for recruitment of research participants, EHRs provide a channel through which researchers may contact patients without prior consent. This "opt-out" methodology expands the reach of information about studies and invitations to participate to a much broader patient population – a tactic that increases and encourages participation by a more diverse population sample (Forsat et al., 2020). In contrast, an "opt-in" methodology would require patients to indicate interest in participating in research to be contacted about opportunities. Furthermore, by using EHRs as tools of outreach to potential study participants, physicians may serve as the first point of contact for the study, providing an endorsement of the study that can help researchers achieve greater success in recruitment and retention.

Many comprehensive EHR systems include patient portals. These components allow for clinicians and researchers to harness the data available through the EHR to conduct proactive outreach to patients for research purposes, in conjunction with local institutional review boards (IRBs). In this way, research teams can ensure the balance of maintaining patient confidentiality and adequate human subjects' protection while offering candidates potential opportunities to engage and learn about clinical research opportunities.

However, alongside the advantages offered by EHRs, researchers must also consider the limitations of these systems. Missing data related to race/ethnicity and other social determinants of health represents a significant problem for researchers seeking to increase participation by historically underrepresented groups (Cook et al., 2021; Grafova & Jarrín, 2021). For example, while race data should be self-reported by patients and entered by clinicians into the EHR, health care staff may misidentify patient race or neglect entirely to record a patient's race and ethnicity in the record. This error may be due to patients choosing not to answer race/ethnicity identification questions or because providers do not ask them. Missing race/ethnicity data leads to the misclassification of patients and, potentially, their exclusion from clinical studies (Yi et al., 2022). Similarly, gender minorities are often classified as either male or female, obscuring important factors that may impact health status and prevention and treatment recommendations. The completeness and accuracy of data within the EHR impact the quality and utility of the algorithms that the EHR builds, based on that data, to identify patients at risk for disease or who may be eligible for participation in a given study.

Some studies, however, have circumvented these problems successfully and provide excellent examples of how to focus on populations of interest. For example, to identify South Asian patients, one study used a selection algorithm that included South Asian surnames; race/ethnicity as defined as Asian Indian, Bangladeshi, Pakistani, or Sri Lankan; and language preference as identified as Bengali, Gujarati, Hindi, Kannada, Kashmiri, Malayalam, Nepali, Pakistani, Punjabi, Sindhi, Sinhalese, Tamil, or Urdu (Beasley et al., 2021). Any one of these three elements was sufficient to identify patients as eligible for participation in the study, allowing researchers to overcome the challenge of missing race/ethnicity data for South Asian patients within the EHR.

Community-based Assets

Employing technology is an important starting point for identifying and engaging older adults in research. However, working with community-based liaisons and partner organizations to support study planning, connect with members of underrepresented populations, and reinforce retention efforts is an equally vital strategy for enhancing the success of community-based clinical research (Ajrouch et al., 2020; Forsat et al., 2020, A. Gilmore-Bykovskyi et al., 2021; Lim et al., 2020; Marshall et al., 2020; Mitchell et al., 2020; Portacolone et al., 2020). This is particularly true with respect to racial and ethnic minoritized and low-income communities. In these settings, frontline health workers – designated in this section as community health workers (CHWs) – play a critical role in conducting outreach, linking individuals to providers, and advising clinicians and researchers regarding appropriate communication strategies, essential logistic concerns, and cultural, linguistic, and socioeconomic factors that may impact study success.

CHWs may be referred to by numerous different terms, including community aides, *promotoras*, lay health workers, peer workers, community health navigators, or patient navigators (CDC, 2014; Love et al., 1997). A fundamental attribute of these individuals is that they are indigenous to the community in which they work – ethnically, linguistically, socioeconomically, and experientially – providing them with a unique understanding of the norms, attitudes, values, and strengths of community members (Giblin, 1989, 1989; Love et al., 1997; Witmer et al., 1995). CHWs bridge the gap between underserved communities and health care providers in efforts to support behavioral change, promote treatment adherence, facilitate access to care, and, more recently, engage community members in research. Key responsibilities of CHWs include bringing in individuals unfamiliar to the health care system, providing cultural linkages, overcoming distrust, supporting patient–provider communication, and increasing the likelihood of patient follow-up.

Nearly three decades ago, a Pew Health Professions Commission report concluded that widespread incorporation of CHWs into the health care system offers unparalleled opportunities to improve the delivery of preventive and primary care to America's diverse communities (Pew Health Professions, 1994) and, today, many programs in the US regularly employ CHWs. Studies using CHW approaches have been found to be effective in improving detection of breast and cervical cancer, childhood immunization rates, smoking cessation, mental health services, timeliness of prenatal care, access to health care, diabetes and hypertension control (CDC, 2014). At the Center for the Study of Asian American Health (CSAAH) at the NYU Grossman School of Medicine, large community-based health disparities research studies have demonstrated that CHW approaches offer a viable and potentially effective strategy to engaging and recruiting individuals from communities already underrepresented in research and build on existing community assets (Islam et al., 2018; Lim et al., 2021; Lopez et al., 2017). The use of community and patient navigators rooted in CHW frameworks has been employed successfully in different settings to engage hard-to-reach and/or underserved populations for diabetes, cardiovascular disease, cancer, mental health, and substance abuse.

Table 5.3 lists specific roles that may be filled effectively by CHWs and the personal characteristics that facilitate the success of individual CHWs functioning in these roles.

Building on these findings, CHW-based approaches for engaging and recruiting older minority and low-income adult patients into aging and AD/ADRD research studies may prove both feasible to implement and culturally acceptable to the communities of interest. Critical to this effort, however, is that CHWs receive extensive training on core competencies including discussing various aspects of clinical research with potential study participants, using motivational interviewing techniques to support health communication messaging about clinical trials, principles of community and participant engagement, and professional and ethical aspects of human subjects' research.

TABLE 5.3 Roles and Characteristics of CHWs

Roles of CHWs	Important Personal Characteristics of CHWs
<ul><li>Educating on health and social issues</li><li>Finding, sharing, and linking resources</li><li>Advocating for participants</li><li>Scheduling and coordinating</li><li>Provide health counseling</li><li>Facilitating communication with service providers due to shared language and cultural characteristics</li><li>Addressing social determinants</li></ul>	<ul><li>A member of that community with a shared history and understanding of the social and cultural context and heightened cultural sensitivities</li><li>Compassionate and empathetic</li><li>Participant-focused</li><li>Good communication skills</li><li>Team player</li><li>Able to establish relationship and identify participant's needs</li><li>Comfortable approaching diverse people/groups and delivering messages – engaging, personable, open</li><li>Good listener</li><li>Good presenter/explainer – comfortable with diverse groups, and sometimes challenging situations</li><li>Comfortable and effective managing conflicts (including intra-family conflicts)</li><li>De-escalation skills</li><li>Work history in community support, care management, clinical research, or related fields</li></ul>

TABLE 5.4 Strategies to Increase Retention of Older Adults in Research

- Maintain and reinforce positive relationships between researchers and participants
- Update participants on study progress and results
- Communicate regularly with participants, care-partners and/or caregivers, and community-based partners
- Solicit feedback from participants regularly; respond to concerns and suggestions
- Provide translations or translators to complete questionnaires and tests on an ongoing basis
- Notify participants before sending follow-up questionnaires
- Demonstrate appreciation for participants
- Provide financial support/incentives to participants and partner organizations throughout the study lifetime
- Work with community health workers and trusted community messengers to highlight the benefits of participating in clinical and community-based research

Importantly, both EHR- and CHW-based approaches contribute not only to recruitment but also retention of older-age participants in research. For example, an automated EHR algorithm may identify participants that miss appointments and prioritize them for follow-up; subsequently, CHWs can reach out to those participants and address their questions, concerns, and other support needs to facilitate their continued participation in the study. A summary of broader retention strategies is presented in Table 5.4.

Testing the recruitment and retention strategies discussed in this chapter using pilot feasibility studies prior to implementing them on a large scale can enhance success and help to avoid pitfalls (Stewart et al., 2020). Ultimately, as increasingly larger community research trials are implemented that prioritize and accommodate the needs of racial and ethnic minoritized and low-income older adults, these more diverse participant populations will be more reflective of the US population at large and these studies will better inform disease prevention and clinical care for older adults in the US.

SUMMARY

By prioritizing linkages with community-based organizations and engaging CHWs, researchers can lay the foundation for long-term success in recruitment of a diverse population of older minoritized and low-income adults in studies. These strategies operationalize the ASK Model and CBPR principles, shifting toward a more inclusive, community-engaged approach to clinical research trials that allows for a broader spectrum of older adults to be included in participant populations. Implementation of these strategies is an urgent priority for clinical researchers, federal agencies, and community-based partner organizations to allow clinical, health services, and public health research and programming to better understand and address the needs of the rapidly growing and diversifying older adult population in the United States.

DISCUSSION QUESTIONS

1. What are the challenges to engaging older populations in clinical trials research?

2. How do participatory and assets-based approaches facilitate engagement and recruitment of minoritized communities in research?

3. Compare community health worker and electronic health record-based strategies for research recruitment.

REFERENCES

Ajrouch, K. J., Vega, I. E., Antonucci, T. C., Tarraf, W., Webster, N. J., & Zahodne, L. B. (2020). Partnering with middle Eastern/Arab American and Latino immigrant communities to increase participation in Alzheimer's disease research. *Ethnicity & Disease*, *30*(Suppl 2), 765–774. https://doi.org/10.18865/ed.30.S2.765

Anderson, R. T., Ory, M., Cohen, S., & McBride, J. S. (2000). Issues of aging and adherence to health interventions. *Controlled Clinical Trials*, *21*(5 Suppl), 171S–83S. https://doi.org/10.1016/s0197-2456(00)00075-1

Ashing-Giwa, K., & Rosales, M. (2012). Recruitment and retention strategies of African American and Latina American breast cancer survivors in a longitudinal psycho-oncology study. *Oncology Nursing Forum*, *39*(5), E434–E442. https://doi.org/10.1188/12.ONF.E434-E442

Beasley, J. M., Ho, J. C., Conderino, S., Thorpe, L. E., Shah, M., Gujral, U. P., Zanowiak, J., & Islam, N. (2021). Diabetes and hypertension among South Asians in New York and Atlanta leveraging hospital electronic health records. *Diabetology & Metabolic Syndrome*, *13*(1), 146. https://doi.org/10.1186/s13098-021-00766-w

Becerra, B. J., Arias, D., & Becerra, M. B. (2017). Low health literacy among immigrant hispanics. *Journal of Racial and Ethnic Health Disparities*, *4*(3), 480–483. https://doi.org/10.1007/s40615-016-0249-5

Bougrab, N., Li, D., Trachtman, H., Sherman, S., Thornton, R., & Langford, A. T. (2019). An electronic health record-based strategy to recruit for a patient advisory council for research: Implications for inclusion. *Journal of Clinical and Translational Science*, *4*(1), 69–72. https://doi.org/10.1017/cts.2019.433

Centers for Disease Control and Prevention. (2014). *States implementing community health worker strategies.* Retrieved from: https://www.cdc.gov/dhdsp/programs/spha/docs/1305_ta_guide_chws.pdf

Centers for Disease Control and Prevention. (2020). What Is Health Literacy? Available at: https://www.cdc.gov/healthliteracy/learn/index.html. Accessed June 14, 2022

Centers for Disease Control and Prevention. (2022). *The U.S. Public Health Service Syphilis Study at Tuskegee.* Available at: https://www.cdc.gov/tuskegee/index.html. Accessed November 16, 2022

Cohen, J. M., Blustein, J., Weinstein, B. E., Dischinger, H., Sherman, S., Grudzen, C., & Chodosh, J. (2017). Studies of physician-patient communication with older patients: How often is hearing loss considered? A systematic literature review. *Journal of the American Geriatrics Society, 65*(8), 1642–1649. https://doi.org/10.1111/jgs.14860

Comis, R. L., Miller, J. D., Aldigé, C. R., Krebs, L., & Stoval, E. (2003). Public attitudes toward participation in cancer clinical trials. *Journal of Clinical Oncology: Official Journal of the American Society of Clinical Oncology, 21*(5), 830–835. https://doi.org/10.1200/JCO.2003.02.105

Cook, L. A., Sachs, J., & Weiskopf, N. G. (2021). The quality of social determinants data in the electronic health record: A systematic review. *Journal of the American Medical Informatics Association: JAMIA, 29*(1), 187–196. https://doi.org/10.1093/jamia/ocab199

D'Alonzo, K. T. (2010). Getting started in CBPR: Lessons in building community partnerships for new researchers. *Nursing Inquiry, 17*(4), 282–288. https://doi.org/10.1111/j.1440-1800.2010.00510.x

Deane, C. S., Phillips, B. E., Smith, K., Steele, A. M., Libretto, T., Statton, S. A., Atherton, P. J., & Etheridge, T. (2020). Challenges and practical recommendations for successfully recruiting inactive, statin-free older adults to clinical trials. *BMC Research Notes, 13*(1), 174. https://doi.org/10.1186/s13104-020-05017-1

Djuric, Z., Ruffin, M. T., 4th, Rapai, M. E., Cornellier, M. L., Ren, J., Ferreri, T. G., Askew, L. M., Sen, A., Brenner, D. E., & Turgeon, D. K. (2012). A Mediterranean dietary intervention in persons at high risk of colon cancer: Recruitment and retention to an intensive study requiring biopsies. *Contemporary Clinical Trials, 33*(5), 881–888. https://doi.org/10.1016/j.cct.2012.05.006

Eborall, H. C., Stewart, M. C., Cunningham-Burley, S., Price, J. F., & Fowkes, F. G. (2011). Accrual and drop out in a primary prevention randomised controlled trial: Qualitative study. *Trials, 12*, 7. https://doi.org/10.1186/1745-6215-12-7

Elliott, M. N., Morrison, P. A., Fremont, A., McCaffrey, D. F., Pantoja, P., & Lurie, N. (2009). Using the Census Bureau's surname list to improve estimates of race/ethnicity and associated disparities. *Health Services and Outcomes Research Method, 9*, 69–83. https://doi.org/10.1007/s10742-009-0047-1

Ford, J. G., Howerton, M. W., Lai, G. Y., Gary, T. L., Bolen, S., Gibbons, M. C., Tilburt, J., Baffi, C., Tanpitukpongse, T. P., Wilson, R. F., Powe, N. R., & Bass, E. B. (2008). Barriers to recruiting underrepresented populations to cancer clinical trials: A systematic review. *Cancer, 112*(2), 228–242. https://doi.org/10.1002/cncr.23157

Forsat, N. D., Palmowski, A., Palmowski, Y., Boers, M., & Buttgereit, F. (2020). Recruitment and retention of older people in clinical research: A systematic literature review. *Journal of the American Geriatrics Society, 68*(12), 2955–2963. https://doi.org/10.1111/jgs.16875

Galea, S., & Tracy, M. (2007). Participation rates in epidemiologic studies. *Annals of Epidemiology, 17*(9), 643–653. https://doi.org/10.1016/j.annepidem.2007.03.013

Giblin, P. T. (1989). Effective utilization and evaluation of indigenous health care workers. *Public Health Rep (Washington D.C.: 1974), 104*(4), 361–368.

Gilmore-Bykovskyi, A., Croff, R., Glover, C. M., Jackson, J. D., Resendez, J., Perez, A., Zuelsdorff, M., Green-Harris, G., & Manly, J. J. (2021). Traversing the aging research and health equity divide: Toward intersectional frameworks of research justice and participation. *The Gerontologist, gnab107*. https://doi.org/10.1093/geront/gnab107

Gilmore-Bykovskyi, A. L., Jin, Y., Gleason, C., Flowers-Benton, S., Block, L. M., Dilworth-Anderson, P., Barnes, L. L., Shah, M. N., & Zuelsdorff, M. (2019). Recruitment and retention of underrepresented populations in Alzheimer's disease research: A systematic review. *Alzheimer's & Dementia (New York, N. Y.), 5*, 751–770. https://doi.org/10.1016/j.trci.2019.09.018

Godbole, N., Kwon, S. C., Beasley, J. M., Roberts, T., Kranick, J., Smilowitz, J., Park, A., Sherman, S. E., Trinh-Shevrin, C., & Chodosh, J. (2022). Assessing equitable inclusion of underrepresented older adults in Alzheimer's Disease, related cognitive disorders, and aging-related research: A scoping review. *The Gerontologist, 63*(6), 1067–1077. https://doi.org/10.1093/geront/gnac060

Grafova, I. B., & Jarrín, O. F. (2021). Beyond black and white: Mapping misclassification of medicare beneficiaries race and ethnicity. *Medical Care Research and Review: MCRR, 78*(5), 616–626. https://doi.org/10.1177/1077558720935733

Hanson, L. C., Gilliam, R., & Lee, T. J. (2010). Successful clinical trial research in nursing homes: The improving decision-making study. *Clinical trials (London, England)*, 7(6), 735–743. https://doi.org/10.1177/1740774510380241

Hasnain-Wynia, R., & Beal, A. C. (2014). Role of the patient-centered outcomes research institute in addressing disparities and engaging patients in clinical research. *Clinical Therapeutics*, 36(5), 619–623. https://doi.org/10.1016/j.clinthera.2014.04.005

Islam, N. S., Wyatt, L. C., Taher, M. D., Riley, L., Tandon, S. D., Tanner, M., Mukherji, B. R., & Trinh-Shevrin, C. (2018). A culturally tailored community health worker intervention leads to improvement in patient-centered outcomes for immigrant patients with type 2 diabetes. *Clinical Diabetes: A Publication of the American Diabetes Association*, 36(2), 100–111. https://doi.org/10.2337/cd17-0068

Israel, B. A., Schulz, A. J., Parker, E. A., & Becker, A. B. (1998). Review of community-based research: Assessing partnership approaches to improve public health. *Annual Review of Public Health*, 19, 173–202. https://doi.org/10.1146/annurev.publhealth.19.1.173

James, D. C., Harville, C., 2nd, Sears, C., Efunbumi, O., & Bondoc, I. (2017). Participation of African Americans in e-Health and m-Health studies: A systematic review. *Telemedicine Journal and E-health: The Official Journal of the American Telemedicine Association*, 23(5), 351–364. https://doi.org/10.1089/tmj.2016.0067

Kamimura, A., Christensen, N., Tabler, J., Ashby, J., & Olson, L. M. (2013). Patients utilizing a free clinic: Physical and mental health, health literacy, and social support. *Journal of Community Health*, 38(4), 716–723. https://doi.org/10.1007/s10900-013-9669-x

Konkel, L. (2015). Racial and ethnic disparities in research studies: The challenge of creating more diverse cohorts. *Environmental Health Perspectives*, 123(12), A297–A302. https://doi.org/10.1289/ehp.123-A297

Kotler, P., & Zaltman, G. (1971). Social marketing: An approach to planned social change. *Journal of Marketing*, 35(3), 3–12. https://doi.org/10.1177/002224297103500302

Langford, A. T. (2020). Health communication and decision making about vaccine clinical trials during a pandemic. *Journal of Health Communication*, 25(10), 780–789. https://doi.org/10.1080/10810730.2020.1864520

Langford, A. T., & Bateman-House, A. (2020). Populations most vulnerable to COVID-19 must be included. *Health Affairs Blog*. June 12, 2020. https://doi.org/10.1377/forefront.20200609.555007

Langford, A. T., Resnicow, K., Dimond, E. P., Denicoff, A. M., Germain, D. S., McCaskill-Stevens, W., Enos, R. A., Carrigan, A., Wilkinson, K., & Go, R. S. (2014). Racial/ethnic differences in clinical trial enrollment, refusal rates, ineligibility, and reasons for decline among patients at sites in the national cancer institute's community cancer centers program. *Cancer*, 120(6), 877–884. https://doi.org/10.1002/cncr.28483

Lim, S., Mohaimin, S., Min, D., Roberts, T., Sohn, Y.-J., Wong, J., Sivanesathurai, R., Kwon, S. C., & Trinh-Shevrin, C. (2020). Alzheimer's disease and its related Dementias among Asian Americans, Native Hawaiians, and Pacific Islanders: A scoping review. *Journal of Alzheimer's Disease: JAD*, 77(2), 523–537. https://doi.org/10.3233/JAD-200509

Lim, S., Wyatt, L. C., Mammen, S., Zanowiak, J. M., Mohaimin, S., Troxel, A. B., Lindau, S. T., Gold, H. T., Shelley, D., Trinh-Shevrin, C., & Islam, N. S. (2021). Implementation of a multi-level community-clinical linkage intervention to improve glycemic control among south Asian patients with uncontrolled diabetes: Study protocol of the DREAM initiative. *BMC Endocrine Disorders*, 21(1), 233. https://doi.org/10.1186/s12902-021-00885-5

Lopez, P. M., Zanowiak, J., Goldfeld, K., Wyka, K., Masoud, A., Beane, S., Kumar, R., Laughlin, P., Trinh-Shevrin, C., Thorpe, L., & Islam, N. (2017). Protocol for project IMPACT (improving millions hearts for provider and community transformation): A quasi-experimental evaluation of an integrated electronic health record and community health worker intervention study to improve hypertension management among South Asian patients. *BMC Health Services Research*, 17(1), 810. https://doi.org/10.1186/s12913-017-2767-1

Love, M. B., Gardner, K., & Legion, V. (1997). Community health workers: Who they are and what they do. *Health Education & Behavior: The Official Publication of the Society for Public Health Education*, 24(4), 510–522. https://doi.org/10.1177/109019819702400409

Mangoni, A. A., Jansen, P. A., & Jackson, S. H. (2013). Under-representation of older adults in pharmacokinetic and pharmacodynamic studies: A solvable problem? *Expert Review of Clinical Pharmacology*, 6(1), 35–39. https://doi.org/10.1586/ecp.12.75

Marshall, L. W., Carrillo, C. A., Reyes, C. E., Thorpe, C. L., Trejo, L., & Sarkisian, C. (2020). Evaluation of recruitment of older adults of color into a community-based chronic disease self-management wellness pathway program in Los Angeles County. *Ethnicity & Disease*, 30(Suppl 2), 735–744. https://doi.org/10.18865/ed.30.S2.735

McDougall, G. J., Jr, Simpson, G., & Friend, M. L. (2015). Strategies for research recruitment and retention of older adults of racial and ethnic minorities. *Journal of Gerontological Nursing*, *41*(5), 14–25. https://doi.org/10.3928/00989134-20150325-01

Meade, C. D., Menard, J. M., Luque, J. S., Martinez-Tyson, D., & Gwede, C. K. (2011). Creating community-academic partnerships for cancer disparities research and health promotion. *Health Promotion Practice*, *12*(3), 456–462. https://doi.org/10.1177/1524839909341035

Michelet, M., Lund, A., & Sveen, U. (2014). Strategies to recruit and retain older adults in intervention studies: A quantitative comparative study. *Archives of Gerontology and Geriatrics*, *59*(1), 25–31. https://doi.org/10.1016/j.archger.2014.03.002

Mitchell, J., Perry, T., Rorai, V., Ilardo, J., Lichtenberg, P. A., & Jackson, J. S. (2020). Building and sustaining a community advisory board of African American older adults as the foundation for volunteer research recruitment and retention in health sciences. *Ethnicity & Disease*, *30*(Suppl 2), 755–764. https://doi.org/10.18865/ed.30.S2.755

Mody, L., Miller, D. K., McGloin, J. M., Freeman, M., Marcantonio, E. R., Magaziner, J., & Studenski, S. (2008). Recruitment and retention of older adults in aging research. *Journal of the American Geriatrics Society*, *56*(12), 2340–2348. https://doi.org/10.1111/j.1532-5415.2008.02015.x

Murray, C. J., Atkinson, C., Bhalla, K., Birbeck, G., Burstein, R., Chou, D., Dellavalle, R., Danaei, G., Ezzati, M., Fahimi, A., Flaxman, D., Foreman, Gabriel, S., Gakidou, E., Kassebaum, N., Khatibzadeh, S., Lim, S., Lipshultz, S. E., London, S., & Lopez, & U.S. Burden of Disease Collaborators. (2013). The state of US health, 1990-2010: Burden of diseases, injuries, and risk factors. *JAMA*, *310*(6), 591–608. https://doi.org/10.1001/jama.2013.13805

National Institute on Aging. (2015). Recruiting Older Adults into Research (ROAR) Toolkit Overview and User Guide. National Institutes of Health. Available at: https://www.nia.nih.gov/research/alzheimers-dementia-outreach-recruitment-engagement-resources/recruiting-older-adults. Accessed June 14, 2022

Normansell, R., Holmes, R., Victor, C., Cook, D. G., Kerry, S., Iliffe, S., Ussher, M., Fox-Rushby, J., Whincup, P., & Harris, T. (2016). Exploring non-participation in primary care physical activity interventions: PACE-UP trial interview findings. *Trials*, *17*, 178. https://doi.org/10.1186/s13063-016-1299-z

Ofstedal, M. B., & Weir, D. R. (2011). Recruitment and retention of minority participants in the health and retirement study. *The Gerontologist*, *51*(Suppl 1), S8–S20. https://doi.org/10.1093/geront/gnq100

Ortman, J. M., Velkoff, V. A., & Hogan, H. (2014). *An Aging Nation: The Older Population in the United States*. Retrieved from: https://www.census.gov/content/dam/Census/library/publications/2014/demo/p25-1140.pdf

Patient Protection and Affordable Care Act. (2010). *Pub. L. No. 111-148 Stat. 124* (March 23, 2010).

Peterson, E. D., Lytle, B. L., Biswas, M. S., & Coombs, L. (2004). Willingness to participate in cardiac trials. *The American Journal of Geriatric Cardiology*, *13*(1), 11–15. https://doi.org/10.1111/j.1076-7460.2004.01709.x

Petrovsky, D. V., Đoàn, L. N., Loizos, M., O'Conor, R., Prochaska, M., Tsang, M., Hopman-Droste, R., Klinedinst, T. C., Mathur, A., Bandeen-Roche, K., van der Willik, O., & Kritchevsky, S. B. (2022). Key recommendations from the 2021 "inclusion of older adults in clinical research" workshop. *Journal of Clinical and Translational Science*, *6*(1), e55. https://doi.org/10.1017/cts.2022.1

Pew Health Professions Commission & University of California San Francisco Center for the Health Professions. (1994). Primary care workforce 2000: Federal policy paper. Pew Health Professions Commission Center for the Health Professions University of California San Francisco.

Polubriaginof, F. C. G., Ryan, P., Salmasian, H., Shapiro, A. W., Perotte, A., Safford, M. M., Hripcsak, G., Smith, S., Tatonetti, N. P., & Vawdrey, D. K. (2019). Challenges with quality of race and ethnicity data in observational databases. *Journal of the American Medical Informatics Association: JAMIA*, *26*(8–9), 730–736. https://doi.org/10.1093/jamia/ocz113

Portacolone, E., Palmer, N. R., Lichtenberg, P., Waters, C. M., Hill, C. V., Keiser, S., Vest, L., Maloof, M., Tran, T., Martinez, P., Guerrero, J., & Johnson, J. K. (2020). Earning the trust of African American communities to increase representation in Dementia research. *Ethnicity & Disease*, *30*(Suppl 2), 719–734. https://doi.org/10.18865/ed.30.S2.719

Rich, M. W., Chyun, D. A., Skolnick, A. H., Alexander, K. P., Forman, D. E., Kitzman, D. W., Maurer, M. S., McClurken, J. B., Resnick, B. M., Shen, W. K., & Tirschwell, D. L., & American Heart Association Older Populations Committee of the Council on Clinical Cardiology, Council on Cardiovascular and Stroke Nursing, Council on Cardiovascular Surgery and Anesthesia, and Stroke Council, & American College of Cardiology; and American Geriatrics Society. (2016). Knowledge gaps in cardiovascular care of the older adult population: A scientific statement from the American Heart Association, American college of cardiology, and American geriatrics society. *Journal of the American College of Cardiology*, *67*(20), 2419–2440. https://www.ahajournals.org/doi/10.1161/CIR.0000000000000380?url_ver=Z39.88-2003&rfr_id=ori:rid:crossref.org&rfr_dat=cr_pub%20%200pubmed

Schron, E. B., Wassertheil-Smoller, S., & Pressel, S. (1997). Clinical trial participant satisfaction: Survey of SHEP enrollees. SHEP Cooperative Research Group. Systolic Hypertension in the Elderly Program. *Journal of the American Geriatrics Society, 45*(8), 934–938. https://doi.org/10.1111/j.1532-5415.1997.tb02962.x

Scott, E., McComb, B., Trachtman, H., Mannon, L., Rosenfeld, P., Thornton, R., Bougrab, N., Sherman, S., & Langford, A. (2019). Knowledge and use of recruitment support tools among study coordinators at an academic medical center: The novel approaches to recruitment planning study. *Contemporary Clinical Trials Communications, 15*, 100424. https://doi.org/10.1016/j.conctc.2019.100424

Shipman, C., Hotopf, M., Richardson, A., Murray, S., Koffman, J., Harding, R., Speck, P., & Higginson, I. J. (2008). The views of patients with advanced cancer regarding participation in serial questionnaire studies. *Palliative Medicine, 22*(8), 913–920. https://doi.org/10.1177/0269216308098087

Sood, J. R., & Stahl, S. M. (2011). Community engagement and the resource centers for minority aging research. *The Gerontologist, 51*(Suppl 1), S5–S7. https://doi.org/10.1093/geront/gnr036

Steinman, L., Hammerback, K., & Snowden, M. (2015). It could be a pearl to you: Exploring recruitment and retention of the program to encourage active, rewarding Lives (PEARLS) With Hard-to-reach populations. *The Gerontologist, 55*(4), 667–676. https://doi.org/10.1093/geront/gnt137

Stenholm, S., Westerlund, H., Head, J., Hyde, M., Kawachi, I., Pentti, J., Kivimäki, M., & Vahtera, J. (2015). Comorbidity and functional trajectories from midlife to old age: The health and retirement study. *The Journals of Gerontology. Series A, Biological Sciences and Medical Sciences, 70*(3), 332–338. https://doi.org/10.1093/gerona/glu113

Stewart, A. L., Nápoles, A. M., Piawah, S., Santoyo-Olsson, J., & Teresi, J. A. (2020). Guidelines for evaluating the feasibility of recruitment in pilot studies of diverse populations: An overlooked but important component. *Ethnicity & Disease, 30*(Suppl 2), 745–754. https://doi.org/10.18865/ed.30.S2.745

Ta Park, V., Grill, J. D., Zhu, J., Nguyen, K., Nam, B., Tsoh, J., Kanaya, A., Vuong, Q., Bang, J., Nguyen, N. C. Y., Cho, I. H., Gallagher-Thompson, D., Hinton, L., & Meyer, O. L. (2021). Asian Americans and Pacific Islanders' perspectives on participating in the CARE recruitment research registry for Alzheimer's disease and related dementias, aging, and caregiving research. *Alzheimer's & Dementia: Translational Research & Clinical Interventions, 7*(1), e12195. https://doi.org/10.1002/trc2.12195

Tanjasiri, S. P., Weiss, J. W., Santos, L., Flores, P., Flores, P., Lacsamana, J. D., Paige, C., Mouttapa, M., Quituqua, L., Taito, P., May, V. T., Tupua, M., Vaikona, E., Vaivao, D., & Vunileva, I. (2015). CBPR-Informed recruitment and retention adaptations in a randomized study of pap testing among Pacific Islanders in Southern California. *Progress in Community Health Partnerships: Research, Education, and Action, 9*(3), 389–396. https://doi.org/10.1353/cpr.2015.0067

Townsley, C. A., Chan, K. K., Pond, G. R., Marquez, C., Siu, L. L., & Straus, S. E. (2006). Understanding the attitudes of the elderly towards enrolment into cancer clinical trials. *BMC Cancer, 6*, 34. https://doi.org/10.1186/1471-2407-6-34

Trinh-Shevrin, C., Islam, N., Tandon, D., Ho-Asjoe, H., & Rey, M. (2007). Using community-based participatory research as a guiding framework for health disparities research centers. *Progress in Community Health Partnerships: Research, Education, and Action, 1*(2), 195–205. https://doi.org/10.1353/cpr.2007.0007

Wallerstein, N., & Duran, B. (2010). Community-based participatory research contributions to intervention research: The intersection of science and practice to improve health equity. *American Journal of Public Health, 100*(Suppl 1), S40–S46. https://doi.org/10.2105/AJPH.2009.184036

Withall, J., Jago, R., & Fox, K. R. (2012). The effect a of community-based social marketing campaign on recruitment and retention of low-income groups into physical activity programmes - a controlled before-and-after study. *BMC Public Health, 12*, 836. https://doi.org/10.1186/1471-2458-12-836

Witham, M. D., & McMurdo, M. E. (2007). How to get older people included in clinical studies. *Drugs & Aging, 24*(3), 187–196. https://doi.org/10.2165/00002512-200724030-00002

Witmer, A., Seifer, S. D., Finocchio, L., Leslie, J., & O'Neil, E. H. (1995). Community health workers: Integral members of the health care work force. *American Journal of Public Health, 85*(8 Pt 1), 1055–1058. https://doi.org/10.2105/ajph.85.8_pt_1.1055

Yi, S. S., Kwon, S. C., Suss, R., Đoàn, L. N., John, I., Islam, N. S., & Trinh-Shevrin, C. (2022). The mutually reinforcing cycle of poor data quality and racialized stereotypes that shapes Asian American health. *Health Affairs (Project Hope), 41*(2), 296–303. https://doi.org/10.1377/hlthaff.2021.01417

Yuval, R., Uziel, K., Gordon, N., Merdler, A., Khader, N., Karkabi, B., Flugelman, M. Y., Halon, D. A., & Lewis, B. S. (2001). Perceived benefit after participating in positive or negative/neutral heart failure trials: The patients' perspective. *European Journal of Heart Failure, 3*(2), 217–223. https://doi.org/10.1016/s1388–9842(00)00151-3

CHAPTER

IMPLEMENTATION SCIENCE APPROACHES TO AGING AND ALZHEIMER'S DISEASE AND ALZHEIMER'S DISEASE-RELATED DEMENTIAS RESEARCH

BETH PRUSACZYK, LISA A. JUCKETT, MATTHEW LEE

LEARNING OBJECTIVES

By the end of this chapter, readers will be able to:

- Identify key implementation science frameworks and theories and how they can be applied to enhance current approaches in aging and Alzheimer's disease and Alzheimer's disease-related dementias (AD/ADRD) research.
- Distinguish implementation science from other types of health services research.

Population Science Methods and Approaches to Aging and Alzheimer's Disease and Related Dementias Research, First Edition. Edited by Chau Trinh-Shevrin.
© 2024 John Wiley & Sons, Inc. Published 2024 by John Wiley & Sons, Inc.

- ▪ Understand how to select appropriate implementation strategies to guide an implementation project or study focused on healthy aging or AD/ADRD.
- ▪ Describe and compare common implementation outcomes.

INTRODUCTION

What Is Implementation Science and Why Do We Need It?

Over the past several decades, there has been significant investment in aging and, specifically, Alzheimer's disease and Alzheimer's disease-related dementias (AD/ADRD) research. The National Institute on Aging's budget continues to be one of the largest among all institutes and centers in the National Institutes of Health, in part due to increases in funding for AD/ADRD research mandated by Congress. As the number of older adults, including those with AD/ADRD, continues to grow, this expanded investment is appropriate as we seek ways to support the health and well-being of older adults, their families, and communities. However, the return-on-investment will be lost and, importantly, we will not make strides in improving the lives of older adults if we do not make an equal investment in translating this funded research into practice.

A commonly-cited statistic is that it takes, on average, 17 years for research findings to reach routine clinical practice (Balas & Boren, 2000). While this single statistic is not definitive, there is widespread agreement that it takes many years – too many – to translate research evidence into real-world change. In addition to preventing us from getting a full return on our research investment, this delay may also be contributing to the disparities we see in care among racial and ethnic minoritized groups and other excluded groups (Baumann & Cabassa, 2020). While we continue to work toward discovering effective clinical treatments and cures for AD/ADRD, we must ensure the most effective behavioral treatments and social services are widely available to people living with dementia and their care partners. These treatments and services are not currently available equally across all groups of people living with dementia. In addition to reducing this disparity, we must also be poised to ensure in the future that those to-be-discovered treatments and cures are disseminated equitably. In other words, closing the research-to-practice gap will benefit all Americans because it will bring to fruition the investment we have made in aging- and AD/ADRD-related research, it will benefit older adults, especially people living with dementia, who deserve evidence-based care and services, and it will benefit historically minoritized and marginalized groups of older adults who have yet to receive evidenced-based care and services on par with the majority.

This research-to-practice gap results from a number of factors at the individual, system, and policy levels. Examples of individual-level factors, or barriers to implementation, include providers' lack of knowledge about research findings and lack of necessary skills or training to deliver new, research-informed care (Karrer et al., 2020). Barriers among patients, people living with dementia, and other non-provider individuals include lack of engagement or positive attitudes toward care (Karrer et al., 2020), especially among racial and ethnic minoritized people (Kenning et al., 2017). At the system or community levels, barriers to research translation include an organization's culture or climate and lack of resources such as personnel and equipment (Karrer et al., 2020). Policy-level barriers include reimbursement policies or quality metrics that do not accommodate new, research-informed care (Prusynski et al., 2021). Additionally, aging-related care and services are often multidisciplinary, involving multiple providers (e.g., medical doctors, nurses, social workers, occupational therapists, case managers, transportation providers) and spanning multiple settings (i.e., inpatient/hospital, outpatient, long-term care, home, and community). This complexity may contribute to confusion as to whose responsibility it is to identify and implement the latest research findings.

The field of *implementation science (IS)* is "the scientific study of methods to promote the systematic uptake of research findings and other evidence-based practices into routine practice, and, hence, to improve the quality and effectiveness of health services" (Eccles & Mittman, 2006). In other words, IS is the scientific study of how we can quickly and effectively close the research-to-practice gap and it is a critical tool in the armamentarium of aging and AD/ADRD-related research. This chapter aims to introduce the reader to IS and provide references and resources for where to find additional information.

Key Terms and Definitions

Before proceeding, it is important to define key terms and concepts within IS. *Dissemination research* is the scientific study of active and focused distribution of information and materials from *evidence-based interventions (EBIs)* to particular audiences through specific channels and using planned strategies. EBIs can include a range of effective health care and prevention strategies, programs, practices, policies, and guidelines that are supported by the best available evidence for routine use (sometimes referred to as "evidence-informed" or "evidence-based" practices). *Dissemination strategies* refer to the *specific mechanisms and channels* used to package and spread information about EBIs to reach key communities and decision-makers in a particular setting, including potential adopters and opinion leaders. In contrast to passive approaches to diffusing information (i.e., expecting practitioners, caregivers, and local champions to identify and digest research publications on their own), dissemination is planned, active, focused, and can be very broad (e.g., mass media campaigns focused toward local policymakers and businesses that highlight the importance of dementia-friendly workplaces) or very narrow (e.g., intensive one-on-one technical assistance) in its scope. Despite the importance of ensuring that research evidence on healthy aging and AD/ADRD is communicated clearly and effectively to key clinical, public health, community, and policy audiences, dissemination remains an understudied domain within IS.

Implementation research refers to the scientific study of using strategies to successfully integrate those EBIs within specific settings in order to improve outcomes and advance population health. These strategies, referred to as *implementation strategies*, are defined as "systematic processes or methods, techniques, activities, and resources that support the adoption, integration, and sustainment of [EBIs] into usual settings" (Rabin & Brownson, 2017). In IS, *adoption* refers to action taken by decision-makers (e.g., organizational or community leaders) to commit to implementing a selected EBI within their setting. Whereas *sustainment* refers to continued EBI use, as intended, over time in ongoing operations (Birken et al., 2020). Relatedly, *sustainability* is the extent to which an EBI can continue to deliver its intended benefits over an extended period of time, particularly after initial funding and support for the effort has ended (Shelton et al., 2018; Shelton & Lee, 2019).

Powell and colleagues (2015) conducted a modified Delphi process with experts to compile and refine implementation strategies and their definitions into a discrete list of 73 strategies referred to as the Expert Recommendations for Implementing Change (ERIC) compilation or compendium. Some examples relevant to aging and AD/ADRD research include discrete actions such as conducting ongoing training related to dementia detection and care, developing or distributing educational materials for dementia caregivers, and developing a formal implementation blueprint for all goals and strategies regarding healthy aging priorities and dementia-related quality metrics. Other implementation strategies focus on generating systems-level action and structural change, such as altering incentive/allowance structures to adopt and implement a comprehensive dementia detection and diagnosis roadmap, changing service sites or physical structures to be older adult- and dementia-friendly, and using data experts and data warehousing techniques across facilities, organizations, and systems to facilitate localized surveillance of aging and AD/ADRD disparities.

Implementation strategies are selected to support successful implementation, which may be assessed by explicitly identifying and assessing *implementation outcomes*, defined as "the effects of deliberate and purposive actions to implement new treatments, practices, and services" (E. Proctor et al., 2011). Some commonly operationalized implementation outcomes include: Feasibility, Acceptability, Appropriateness, Adoption, Fidelity, Dose, Reach/Penetration, Sustainability, and Costs. These outcomes will be discussed later in the chapter.

Importantly, implementation outcomes must be understood as distinct from intervention outcomes at the clinical, treatment, behavioral, or service levels. However, they are also necessary precursors to intervention success: failing to achieve implementation outcomes will result in poor intervention outcomes. For example, if the selected implementation strategies do not achieve sufficient and equitable reach/penetration within a setting, it is likely that the overall change effort will not be successful, particularly in addressing dementia disparities.

EBIs are often developed and evaluated in an organization or community in which resources and capacity differ from the context in which the current change effort is taking place. In these instances, *adaptation* may be necessary to meaningfully tailor the EBI to better meet local needs and context. A key domain in IS, adaptation is defined by Stirman and colleagues (2019) as "the process of thoughtful and deliberate alteration to the design or delivery of an intervention, with the goal of improving its fit or effectiveness in a given context." *Cultural adaptation*, more specifically, refers to modifications that pay explicit attention to the importance of cultural patterns, meanings, and values within the community context and seeks to integrate both observable and cognitive aspects of a local culture into intervention content (Barrera et al., 2013; Lee & Kwon, 2022). As defined by Bernal and colleagues (2009), cultural adaptation is "the systematic modification of an evidence-based treatment or intervention protocol to consider language, culture, and context in such a way that it is compatible with the client [and community's] cultural patterns, meanings, and values."

The concepts of *scaling-up* and *scaling-out* are also relevant to implementation research focused on healthy aging and AD/ADRD, particularly since best practices and effective approaches will likely spread to additional similar settings (scale-up) – e.g., to additional clinics within the same health system – or even to entirely new areas (scale-out) – e.g., to clinics and health systems in other regions. As defined by Aarons and colleagues (2017), *scale-up* is "the deliberate effort to broaden the delivery of an EBI with the intention of reaching larger numbers of a target audience" whereas *scale-out* is "an extension of scale-up and uniquely refers to the deliberate use of strategies to implement, test, improve, and sustain an EBI as it is delivered to new populations and/or through new delivery systems that differ from those in effectiveness trials."

Lastly, *hybrid designs* in IS involve the joint study of effectiveness *and* implementation together to facilitate timelier uptake of key interventions and generate more relevant information for future scale-up and have become increasingly common in implementation research (Curran et al., 2012). Hybrid effectiveness-implementation designs can span a continuum of three types: *Type I Hybrid Designs* primarily focus on testing the effectiveness of the EBI while also collecting data on implementation as a secondary outcome, *Type II Hybrid Designs* simultaneously test both the effectiveness of the EBI and the implementation strategies and place an equal emphasis on both, and *Type III Hybrid Designs* focus primarily on testing the effectiveness of implementation strategies while collecting data on intervention effectiveness as a secondary outcome.

How Does IS Differ from Other Types of Research and Operational Activities?

For those who are new to IS, it is often valuable to situate IS within the larger field of health services research (HSR) and differentiate it from other types of HSR. This is helpful not only for learning IS but also for understanding how IS fits along the research translation continuum.

A well-known research translation framework first conceptualized by the Institute of Medicine (IOM) and then built upon by additional researchers characterizes research translation along a continuum (Fort et al., 2017). In this framework, "T0" research is basic, preclinical research; "T1" research is focused on translating research from T0 to humans (e.g., Phase 1 clinical trials); and "T2" moves research from humans to patients (e.g., Phase 2 and Phase 3 clinical trials). It is in the next phases – "T3" and "T4" – where IS is often placed. T3 research moves from patients into practice and T4 is focused on outcomes and effectiveness at the population level.

Using this framework, IS begins once research has been thoroughly tested and found to be effective. However, increasingly, this framework is not thought to be linear and, importantly, there are calls for research being conducted in the T1 and T2 phases to incorporate IS principles so that it is more likely to be translated from T2 to T3 and T4. For example, there is key implementation information, such as barriers to implementation, that can be collected during Phase 2 and Phase 3 clinical trials that can inform how the intervention is delivered at the population level. Therefore, while IS specifically focuses on taking existing research evidence (i.e., research that has been thoroughly studied in earlier phases) and scientifically studying its adoption into routine practice, researchers at all stages should be attuned to the translation gap mentioned earlier and incorporate IS principles into their work to ensure it reaches the populations it is intended to serve.

Other types of research or operational activities that are useful to differentiate from IS include comparative effectiveness research (CER) and quality improvement (QI). The IOM defines CER as research that "compares the benefits and harms of alternative methods to prevent, diagnose, treat, and monitor a clinical condition, or to improve the delivery of care" (Sox & Greenfield, 2009). Similar to IS, CER involves comparing interventions that have *already been shown to be effective*. Additionally, CER is also conducted among participants in real-world clinical settings (i.e., as opposed to human subjects in controlled, research trials). Therefore, like IS, CER is considered a T3 or T4 field of research, beginning once efficacy and effectiveness have been established. However, CER differs from IS in that the primary outcome of CER is effectiveness and the primary outcomes in IS are the uptake, adoption, implementation, acceptability, etc., of the intervention. Thus, in IS, researchers are studying what strategies or actions increase those IS outcomes rather than examining the effectiveness of the interventions, unlike CER researchers.

QI is not typically considered research because it is not focused on creating generalizable knowledge and, instead, is driven by a specific quality concern or gap (Bauer & Kirchner, 2020). A QI project is also often focused on a single setting – e.g., a single clinic or hospital – and the goal is to intervene and measure improvement in that setting for that specific quality metric. It is understandable, then, that many QI projects implement existing EBIs that have been identified to improve the specific quality concern of that project. However, similar to CER, the outcomes often differ between QI and IS. QI is focused on measuring quality indicators (e.g., length of stay, infection rates, wait times) while IS is focused on uptake, adoption, etc. This distinct focus of IS differentiates it from other types of research or operational activities and highlights its unique and important role in improving the lives of individuals across the lifespan.

Key IS Theories and Frameworks

Implementation scientists have developed a wide array of theories and frameworks to grow the field. These theories and frameworks have been applied to identify relevant contextual factors, potential barriers, and facilitators associated with adoption, implementation, and sustainment, as well as to guide planning, measurement, and evaluation in implementation studies.

Some frameworks have focused on compiling and organizing commonly-studied theories and factors across implementation studies. For example, the Theoretical Domains Framework (TDF) groups constructs from behavior and behavior change theories into 14 domains and has been widely used by health care systems to explain implementation problems and inform implementation studies (Atkins et al., 2017; Cane et al., 2012; Michie et al., 2005). Similarly, the Consolidated Framework for Implementation Research (CFIR) describes 39 theoretical constructs across five domains: 1) outer context, 2) inner context, 3) implementation processes, 4) intervention characteristics, and 5) characteristics of individuals and has been widely used to plan for and evaluate the impact of these constructs on implementation success (Damschroder et al., 2009). For example, Morgan and colleagues (2019) recently used the CFIR to guide data collection and analysis for a longitudinal (2.5 year) process evaluation of a participatory effort to codesign and implement an evidence-based interdisciplinary rural primary health care memory clinic in the Saskatchewan province of Canada. Using this approach, they were able to identify barriers and facilitators impacting the development and implementation of a rural-specific strategy for dementia assessment and management in primary health care.

Other frameworks highlight important domains or phases within IS and describe common and unique factors within each one. For example, the EPIS framework by Aarons and colleagues (2011) highlights four iterative phases that align with the implementation process: Exploration, Preparation/Adoption, Implementation, and Sustainment. Similarly, Koh and colleagues (Koh et al., 2020) introduced five key domains within D&I science: Context Assessment/EBI selection, Dissemination, Adaptation, Implementation, and Sustainability.

Another IS framework that has demonstrated great versatility in informing intervention and implementation design, planning, and evaluation is the RE-AIM framework, which describes five phases: Reach, Effectiveness, Adoption, Implementation, and Maintenance (Glasgow et al., 2019, 1999). Originally developed to facilitate transparency in reporting, RE-AIM has become one of the most widely used frameworks in IS. Extensions of RE-AIM have also been widely applied, notably the PRISM (Practical Robust Implementation and Sustainability Model) to support pragmatic application and identify contextual factors across community and clinical settings (Feldstein & Glasgow, 2008; McCreight et al., 2019). In a scoping review of implementation research in dementia care, Lourida and colleagues (2017) found that only 38 of the 88 studies included in the final review reported using a theory or framework, with RE-AIM being the most commonly cited framework (n = 5).

Efforts have been made to help practitioners and researchers navigate this landscape, particularly those who are new to the field. For example, Nilsen (2015) organized and proposed a taxonomy of five different categories of theories and frameworks in IS: 1) process models, 2) determinants frameworks, 3) classic theories, 4) implementation theories, and 5) evaluation frameworks. Additionally, Tabak and colleagues (2012) reviewed commonly cited models in IS and identified, analyzed, and categorized 61 models across three variables: 1) construct flexibility, 2) focus on dissemination and/or implementation activities, and 3) socioecological level(s). Stemming from the Tabak et al. review and another one by Mitchell and colleagues (2010), an interactive online tool was recently created by a collaborative from the University of Colorado, Denver, Washington University in St. Louis, and University of California, San Diego for practitioners and researchers to select which model or models may best suit their practice problem or research question and is available at https://dissemination-implementation.org.

Implementation Strategies

Theories and frameworks used to guide IS work are also critically important to inform researchers' selection of *implementation strategies*. As defined earlier, implementation strategies are the methods or approaches used to facilitate the uptake of effective interventions and programs into real-world practice (Proctor et al., 2013). Key classifications of implementation strategies include the Effective Practice and Organisation of Care (EPOC) taxonomy (Cochrane, 2015) and the Expert Recommendations for Implementing Change (ERIC) taxonomy (Powell et al., 2015). The ERIC taxonomy, referenced earlier, provides detailed explanations of over 70 strategies developed to promote evidence implementation. Examples of these strategies include identifying early evidence adopters, conducting local needs assessments, obtaining client and family feedback, altering incentive structures, and conducting ongoing training.

While implementation taxonomies serve as helpful resources in the design of IS studies, prior to strategy selection, researchers must *first* carefully evaluate the complex barriers and facilitators that may influence implementation activities across practice contexts (e.g., skilled nursing facilities, community-based organizations) (Elwy et al., 2020). Once identified, researchers can then select and develop strategies designed to overcome implementation barriers (e.g., lack of administrative support) and leverage implementation facilitators (e.g., strong practitioner buy-in).

Though implementation strategies have been found effective for promoting the uptake of EBIs (Goorts et al., 2021), the overall body of evidence on strategy effectiveness is rather mixed, which may be attributed partially to the lack of clarity on how researchers should approach implementation strategy selection (Powell et al., 2019). Fortunately, the process of selecting and developing such strategies has been elucidated in recent years through advancements in IS methodologies. Examples of these strategy selection methods include concept mapping, intervention mapping, group model building, and conjoint analysis (Powell et al., 2017). *Concept mapping* is a mixed-methods approach that requires heavy involvement of stakeholders in a combination of brainstorming, sorting, and rating tasks on a topic of inquiry. *Intervention mapping* is a multistep process that includes the completion of a needs assessment, the identification of project objectives and implementation strategies to achieve such objectives, the design of implementation strategies, and the ongoing assessment of strategy effectiveness (Fernandez et al., 2019). *Group model building* leverages stakeholder feedback to identify a problem of interest – such as the inadequate use of an EBI – and design potential implementation strategies to address that problem. A key feature of group model building includes the development of a mathematical simulation model to evaluate the extent to which the proposed implementation strategies impact the problem of interest. Lastly, *conjoint analysis* includes the convening of stakeholders who are asked to rate their likelihood of using a combination of implementation strategies to facilitate evidence uptake (Powell et al., 2017).

Given that the unique needs of clients, practitioners, organizations, and systems vary widely, it is difficult to establish consensus on the types of implementation strategies that are most effective across practice contexts. However, we do know that multifaceted implementation strategies appear to be supported by stronger evidence as compared to singular or discrete implementation strategies (Goorts et al., 2021). Specific to AD/ADRD research, Baker et al. (Baker et al., 2019) deployed a combination of strategies to support the implementation of music therapy for people living with dementia. Strategies included the ongoing training of clinicians, the provision of feedback to clinicians after auditing music therapy sessions, and the development of educational materials. Further, the combination of interactive trainings and the appointment of pain "champions" promoted the adoption of pain management guidelines within dementia care settings (Brunkert et al., 2021).

Implementation Outcomes

Implementation strategies typically are deemed "effective" if they lead to improvements in *implementation outcomes*. While efficacy and effectiveness in intervention research are often established through improvements in individual-level outcomes, the efficacy and effectiveness of implementation strategies are measured by evaluating changes in implementation outcomes that represent perspectives, attitudes, and behaviors of clients, clinicians, organizations, and/or systems (Proctor et al., 2009).

Just as implementation theories and frameworks can guide the implementation process and the identification of implementation determinants (e.g., barriers and facilitators), theories and frameworks can also inform the evaluation of implementation outcomes. For instance, the aforementioned RE-AIM (Reach, Effectiveness, Adoption, Implementation, and Maintenance) framework can be applied to evaluate EBI implementation. *Reach* refers to the proportion of eligible individuals who receive an intervention. *Effectiveness* represents the positive and negative consequences of an intervention that pertain to physiologic, behavioral, and/or physical outcomes. *Adoption* is considered the proportion of clinics, facilities, or communities that use an intervention of interest. *Implementation* refers to the degree to which a program or intervention is delivered by clinicians or organizations as it was originally intended and also refers to clients' level of adherence to program components. Lastly, *Maintenance* refers to the extent to which an intervention is routinely used to impact the health of individuals or communities over time (Glasgow et al., 1999).

Relatedly, the Implementation Outcomes Framework is composed of the following eight outcomes: acceptability, adoption, appropriateness, cost, feasibility, fidelity, penetration, and sustainability. *Acceptability* can be measured at the client or provider level and represents satisfaction with a particular intervention and its components. *Adoption* is conceptualized as the "uptake" of an intervention in practice; *appropriateness* is the perceived fit of an intervention given the needs of the client, provider, or setting; whereas *feasibility* is the actual fit or utility of an intervention for everyday use. Similar to the "Implementation" dimension of the RE-AIM model, *fidelity* is the extent to which an intervention is delivered as it was originally intended. *Cost* refers to cost savings, cost-effectiveness, and/or cost-benefits and is an understudied though crucial outcome in IS research. *Penetration* is the level of spread, or reach, of an intervention; and *sustainability* is the degree to which an intervention can be sustained in practice over time (E. Proctor et al., 2011). Instruments such as the Acceptability of Implementation Measure, the Intervention Outcome Measure, and the Feasibility of Implementation Measure were directly informed by the IOF and can be used to assess the implementability of EBIs or can serve to measure the effectiveness of implementation strategies (Weiner et al., 2017).

In AD/ADRD research, Proctor et al.'s IOF guided the evaluation of the Care of People with dementia in their Environments (COPE) intervention implemented in dementia care contexts in Australia. Specifically, COPE developers deployed a combination of implementation strategies (e.g., develop educational materials, build stakeholder buy-in, monitor quality) to increase adoption and fidelity of COPE by occupational therapists and nurses across 17 dementia care organizations (Clemson et al., 2021). Alternatively, the RE-AIM framework was used to inform the collection and analysis of qualitative data representing stakeholder (i.e., social workers, nursing staff, administrators) perceptions of implementing the Evidence Integration Triangle for Behavioral and Psychological Symptoms of Distress in Dementia (EIT-4-BPSD) strategy in 21 nursing homes across Maryland and Pennsylvania (Behrens et al., 2021).

SUMMARY

The implementation research process can be summarized through a research logic model (Figure 6.1), which begins with an evidence-based practice and includes identifying factors that will influence its implementation, designing the best approach to address these factors, and assessing outcomes at the implementation, service, and client levels. All providers and researchers can incorporate these IS concepts into their research and practice, whether that is by designing their interventions with implementation and sustainability in mind or

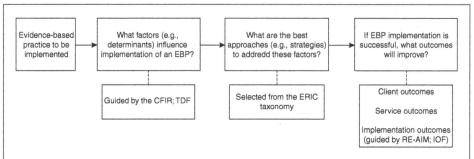

FIGURE 6.1 *Implementation Research Logic Model for AD/ADRD research. Adapted from Smith et al. (2020). EBP = evidence-based practice, referring to interventions, programs, guidelines, assessments, and/or innovations. CFIR = Consolidated Framework for Implementation Research; TDF = Theoretical Domains Framework; ERIC = Expert Recommendations for Implementing Change taxonomy; RE-AIM = Reach Effectiveness Adoption Implementation Maintenance framework; IOF = Implementation Outcomes Framework*

designing QI or clinical workflows using IS strategies. This is critical if we are to see significant improvement in the lives of older adults, especially those with AD/ADRD. It is not enough to develop new treatments and interventions. We must ensure those treatments and interventions equitably reach and impact communities and do not end up only as words in an academic article. IS is a primary way we can do this.

DISCUSSION QUESTIONS

1. How might you incorporate concepts from implementation science into your current aging or AD/ADRD research? Clinical or community-based care?

2. Given your specific population, setting, or problem of interest, what possible implementation strategies do you think would be appropriate to use to overcome implementation barriers?

3. What implementation outcomes are most applicable to your current research or practices?

REFERENCES

Aarons, G. A., Hurlburt, M., & Horwitz, S. M. C. (2011). Advancing a conceptual model of evidence-based practice implementation in public service sectors. *Administration and Policy in Mental Health and Mental Health Services Research*, *38*(1). https://doi.org/10.1007/s10488-010-0327-7

Aarons, G. A., Sklar, M., Mustanski, B., Benbow, N., & Brown, C. H. (2017). "Scaling-out" evidence-based interventions to new populations or new health care delivery systems. *Implementation Science*, *12*(1). https://doi.org/10.1186/s13012-017-0640-6

Atkins, L., Francis, J., Islam, R., & Michie, S. (2017). A guide to using the theoretical domains framework of behaviour change to investigate implementation problems. *Implementation Science, 12*(1). https://doi.org/10.1186/s13012-017-0605-9

Baker, F. A., Tamplin, J., Clark, I. N., Lee, Y. E. C., Geretsegger, M., & Gold, C. (2019). Treatment fidelity in a music therapy multi-site cluster randomized controlled trial for people living with dementia: The middel project intervention fidelity protocol. *Journal of Music Therapy, 56*(2). https://doi.org/10.1093/jmt/thy023

Balas, E. A., & Boren, S. A. (2000). Managing clinical knowledge for health care improvement. *Yearbook of Medical Informatics, 09*(01). https://doi.org/10.1055/s-0038-1637943

Barrera, M., Jr, Castro, F. G., Strycker, L. A., & Toobert, D. J. (2013). Cultural adaptations of behavioral health interventions: A progress report. *Journal of Consulting and Clinical Psychology, 81*(2), 196–205. https://doi.org/10.1037/a0027085

Bauer, M. S., & Kirchner, J. A. (2020). Implementation science: What is it and why should I care? *Psychiatry Research*. https://doi.org/10.1016/j.psychres.2019.04.025

Baumann, A. A., & Cabassa, L. J. (2020). Reframing implementation science to address inequities in healthcare delivery. *BMC Health Services Research, 20*(1). https://doi.org/10.1186/s12913-020-4975-3

Behrens, L., Boltz, M., Riley, K., Eshraghi, K., Resnick, B., Galik, E., Ellis, J., Kolanowski, A., & Van Haitsma, K. (2021). Process evaluation of an implementation study in dementia care (EIT-4-BPSD): Stakeholder perspectives. *BMC Health Services Research, 21*(1), 1006. https://doi.org/10.1186/s12913-021-07001-2

Bernal, G., Jiménez-Chafey, M. I., & Domenech Rodríguez, M. M. (2009). Cultural adaptation of treatments: A resource for considering culture in evidence-based practice. *Professional Psychology: Research and Practice, 40*(4). https://doi.org/10.1037/a0016401

Birken, S. A., Haines, E. R., Hwang, S., Chambers, D. A., Bunger, A. C., & Nilsen, P. (2020). Advancing understanding and identifying strategies for sustaining evidence-based practices: A review of reviews. *Implementation Science*. https://doi.org/10.1186/s13012-020-01040-9

Brunkert, T., Simon, M., & Zúñiga, F. (2021). Use of pain management champions to enhance guideline implementation by care workers in nursing homes. *Worldviews on Evidence-Based Nursing, 18*(2). https://doi.org/10.1111/wvn.12499

Cane, J., O'Connor, D., & Michie, S. (2012). Validation of the theoretical domains framework for use in behaviour change and implementation research. *Implementation Science, 7*(1). https://doi.org/10.1186/1748-5908-7-37

Clemson, L., Laver, K., Rahja, M., & Gitlin, L. N. (2021). Implementing a reablement intervention, "care of people with dementia in their environments (COPE)": A hybrid implementation-effectiveness study. *Gerontologist, 61*(6). https://doi.org/10.1093/geront/gnaa105

Cochrane. (2015). Effective practice and organisation of care (EPOC). EPOC Taxonomy.

Curran, G. M., Bauer, M., Mittman, B., Pyne, J. M., & Stetler, C. (2012). Effectiveness-implementation hybrid designs: Combining elements of clinical effectiveness and implementation research to enhance public health impact. *Medical Care, 50*, 217–226. https://doi.org/10.1097/MLR.0b013e3182408812

Damschroder, L. J., Aron, D. C., Keith, R. E., Kirsh, S. R., Alexander, J. A., & Lowery, J. C. (2009). Fostering implementation of health services research findings into practice: A consolidated framework for advancing implementation science. *Implementation Science: IS, 4*, 50. https://doi.org/10.1186/1748-5908-4-50

Eccles, M. P., & Mittman, B. S. (2006). Welcome to implementation science. *Implementation Science, 1*(1), 1. https://doi.org/10.1186/1748-5908-1-1

Elwy, A. R., Wasan, A. D., Gillman, A. G., & Greco, C. M. (2020). Using formative evaluation methods to improve clinical implementation efforts: Description and an example. *Psychiatry Research, 283*. https://doi.org/10.1016/j.psychres.2019.112532

Feldstein, A. C., & Glasgow, R. E. (2008). A practical, robust implementation and sustainability model (PRISM) for integrating research findings into practice. *Joint Commission Journal on Quality and Patient Safety, 34*(4), 228–243. https://doi.org/10.1016/s1553-7250(08)34030-6

Fernandez, M. E., ten Hoor, G. A., van Lieshout, S., & Kok, G. (2019). Implementation mapping: Using intervention mapping to develop implementation strategies. *Frontiers in Public Health, 7*(JUN). https://doi.org/10.3389/fpubh.2019.00158

Fort, D. G., Herr, T. M., Shaw, P. L., Gutzman, K. E., & Starren, J. B. (2017). Mapping the evolving definitions of translational research. *Journal of Clinical and Translational Science, 1*(1). https://doi.org/10.1017/cts.2016.10

Glasgow, R. E., Harden, S. M., Gaglio, B., & Estabrooks, P. A. (2019). RE-AIM planning and evaluation framework: Adapting to new science and practice with a 20-year review. *Frontiers in Public Health*. https://doi.org/10.3389/fpubh.2019.00064

Glasgow, R. E., Vogt, T. M., & Boles, S. M. (1999). Evaluating the public health impact of health promotion interventions: The RE-AIM framework. *American Journal of Public Health*. https://doi.org/10.2105/AJPH.89.9.1322

Goorts, K., Dizon, J., & Milanese, S. (2021). The effectiveness of implementation strategies for promoting evidence informed interventions in allied healthcare: A systematic review. *BMC Health Services Research*, *21*(1). https://doi.org/10.1186/s12913-021-06190-0

Karrer, M., Hirt, J., Zeller, A., & Saxer, S. (2020). What hinders and facilitates the implementation of nurse-led interventions in dementia care? A scoping review. *BMC Geriatrics*, *20*(1). https://doi.org/10.1186/s12877-020-01520-z

Kenning, C., Daker-White, G., Blakemore, A., Panagioti, M., & Waheed, W. (2017). Barriers and facilitators in accessing dementia care by ethnic minority groups: A meta-synthesis of qualitative studies. *BMC Psychiatry*, *17*(1). https://doi.org/10.1186/s12888-017-1474-0

Koh, S., Lee, M., Brotzman, L. E., & Shelton, R. C. (2020). An orientation for new researchers to key domains, processes, and resources in implementation science. *Translational Behavioral Medicine*, *10*(1), 179–185. https://doi.org/10.1093/tbm/iby095

Lee, M., & Kwon, S. C. (Forthcoming 2022). Chapter 7: Participatory dissemination & implementation research in community settings. In: C. Trinh-Shevrin, N. Islam, S. Yi, & S. Kwon. (Eds.), Applied population health approaches for Asian American communities. Wiley.

Lourida, I., Abbott, R. A., Rogers, M., & Thompson Coon, J. (2017). Dissemination and implementation research in dementia care: A systematic scoping review and evidence map. *BMC Geriatrics*. https://doi.org/10.1186/s12877-017-0528-y

McCreight, M. S., Rabin, B. A., Glasgow, R. E., & Battaglia, C. T. (2019). Using the practical, robust implementation and sustainability model (PRISM) to qualitatively assess multilevel contextual factors to help plan, implement, evaluate, and disseminate health services programs. *Translational Behavioral Medicine*, *9*(6). https://doi.org/10.1093/tbm/ibz085

Michie, S., Johnston, M., Abraham, C., Lawton, R., Parker, D., & Walker, A. (2005). Making psychological theory useful for implementing evidence based practice: A consensus approach. *Quality and Safety in Health Care*, *14*. https://doi.org/10.1136/qshc.2004.011155

Mitchell, S. A., Fisher, C. A., Hastings, C. E., Silverman, L. B., & Wallen, G. R. (2010). A thematic analysis of theoretical models for translational science in nursing: Mapping the field. *Nursing Outlook*, *58*(6). https://doi.org/10.1016/j.outlook.2010.07.001

Morgan, D., Kosteniuk, J., O'Connell, M. E., & Sauter, K. (2019). Barriers and facilitators to development and implementation of a rural primary health care intervention for dementia: A process evaluation. *BMC Health Services Research*, *19*(1), N.PAG–N.PAG. https://doi.org/10.1186/s12913-019-4548-5

Nilsen, P. (2015). Making sense of implementation theories, models and frameworks. *Implement Science*, *10*, 53. https://doi.org/10.1186/s13012-015-0242-0

Powell, B. J., Beidas, R. S., Lewis, C. C., & Mandell, D. S. (2017). Methods to improve the selection and tailoring of implementation strategies. *Journal of Behavioral Health Services and Research*, *44*(2). https://doi.org/10.1007/s11414-015-9475-6

Powell, B. J., Fernandez, M. E., Williams, N. J., & Weiner, B. J. (2019). Enhancing the impact of implementation strategies in healthcare: A research agenda. *Frontiers in Public Health*, *7*(JAN). https://doi.org/10.3389/fpubh.2019.00003

Powell, B. J., Waltz, T. J., Chinman, M. J., & Kirchner, J. A. E. (2015). A refined compilation of implementation strategies: Results from the expert recommendations for implementing change (ERIC) project. *Implementation Science*, *10*(1). https://doi.org/10.1186/s13012-015-0209-1

Proctor, E., Silmere, H., Raghavan, R., … Hensley, M. (2011). Outcomes for implementation research: Conceptual distinctions, measurement challenges, and research agenda. *Administration and Policy in Mental Health and Mental Health Services Research*, *38*(2). https://doi.org/10.1007/s10488-010-0319-7

Proctor, E. K., Landsverk, J., Aarons, G., Chambers, D., Glisson, C., & Mittman, B. (2009). Implementation research in mental health services: An emerging science with conceptual, methodological, and training challenges. *Administration and Policy in Mental Health and Mental Health Services Research*, *36*(1). https://doi.org/10.1007/s10488-008-0197-4

Proctor, E. K., Powell, B. J., & McMillen, J. C. (2013). Implementation strategies: Recommendations for specifying and reporting. *Implementation Science*, *8*(1). https://doi.org/10.1186/1748-5908-8-139

Prusynski, R. A., Leland, N. E., Frogner, B. K., Leibbrand, C., & Mroz, T. M. (2021). Therapy staffing in skilled nursing facilities declined after implementation of the patient-driven payment model. *Journal of the American Medical Directors Association, 22*(10). https://doi.org/10.1016/j.jamda.2021.04.005

Rabin, B. A., & Brownson, R. C. (2017). Terminology for dissemination and implementation research. In: R.C. Brownson, G. A. Colditz, & E. K. Proctor. (Eds.), Dissemination and Implementation Research in Health: Translating Science to Practice, (Second ed). Oxford Academic. https://doi.org/10.1093/oso/9780190683214.003.0002.

Shelton, R. C., Cooper, B. R., & Stirman, S. W. (2018). The sustainability of evidence-based interventions and practices in public health and health care. *Annual Review of Public Health, 39*. https://doi.org/10.1146/annurev-publhealth-040617-014731

Shelton, R. C., & Lee, M. (2019). Sustaining evidence-based interventions and policies: Recent innovations and future directions in implementation science. *American Journal of Public Health, 109*(S2), S132–S134. https://doi.org/10.2105/AJPH.2018.304913

Smith, J. D., Li, D. H., & Rafferty, M. R. (2020). The Implementation Research Logic Model: A method for planning, executing, reporting, and synthesizing implementation projects. *Implementation Science: IS, 15*(1), 84. https://doi.org/10.1186/s13012-020-01041-8

Sox, H. C., & Greenfield, S. (2009). Comparative effectiveness research: A report from the institute of medicine. *Annals of Internal Medicine, 151*(3), 203–205. https://doi.org/10.7326/0003-4819-151-3-200908040-00125

Stirman, S. W., Baumann, A. A., & Miller, C. J. (2019). The FRAME: An expanded framework for reporting adaptations and modifications to evidence-based interventions. *Implementation Science, 14*(1). https://doi.org/10.1186/s13012-019-0898-y

Tabak, R. G., Khoong, E. C., Chambers, D. A., & Brownson, R. C. (2012). Bridging research and practice: Models for dissemination and implementation research. *American Journal of Preventive Medicine, 43*(3), 337–350. https://doi.org/10.1016/j.amepre.2012.05.024

Weiner, B. J., Lewis, C. C., Stanick, C., & Halko, H. (2017). Psychometric assessment of three newly developed implementation outcome measures. *Implementation Science, 12*(1). https://doi.org/10.1186/s13012-017-0635-3

CHAPTER

GROUP MODEL BUILDING TO PROMOTE PUBLIC HEALTH RESEARCH AND ACTION

RACHEL L. THOMPSON, DAVID W. LOUNSBURY, MIRNOVA E. CEÏDE, TERRY T-K HUANG, NASIM S. SABOUNCHI

LEARNING OBJECTIVES

By the end of this chapter, readers will be able to:

- Apply general methods in group model building (GMB) as a strategy to build public health partnerships for research and action in Alzheimer's disease and Alzheimer's disease-related dementias (AD/ADRD).

- Identify priorities for public health research and action in AD/ADRD.

- Synthesize extant knowledge about the potential for evidence-based psychosocial interventions as a means to slow cognitive decline in persons with AD/ADRD.

Population Science Methods and Approaches to Aging and Alzheimer's Disease and Related Dementias Research, First Edition. Edited by Chau Trinh-Shevrin.
© 2024 John Wiley & Sons, Inc. Published 2024 by John Wiley & Sons, Inc.

INTRODUCTION

The global burden of Alzheimer's disease and Alzheimer's disease-related dementias (AD/ADRD) is substantial and expected to rise in the coming decades due to population growth, specifically growth of the aging population. The 2019 Global Burden of Disease study estimated that 57.4 million people were living with dementia in 2019 and projected that number to increase to 152.8 million in 2050 (Nichols et al., 2022). Management of AD/ADRD constitutes significant costs to individuals affected by the disease as well as broader society. Currently, the United States spends $593 billion on AD/ADRD management annually, which includes $321 billion in direct care costs and $272 billion in unpaid dementia caregiving (Alzheimer's Disease Facts and Figures, 2022).

Our current understanding of causes of AD/ADRD is growing rapidly, as is our understanding of evidence-based clinical interventions to treat and manage these conditions. Billions of dollars have been invested in research and development of drugs to treat AD in past decades; however, these efforts have been largely unsuccessful, producing only a handful of drugs which merely treat the symptoms of AD rather than affect the underlying biological causes of the disease (Cummings et al., 2022). Failure to develop efficacious drugs to treat AD/ADRD and the rising costs of managing AD/ADRD morbidity demand that the focus of research efforts be shifted toward identifying non-pharmacologic interventions to target modifiable causes of AD/ADRD, especially considering that less than 1% of AD cases are caused by deterministic genes (Alzheimer's Association, 2022).

The *Lancet* commission on dementia prevention, intervention, and care has identified 12 modifiable risk factors that could prevent or delay up to 40% of dementias: education, hypertension, hearing impairment, smoking, obesity, depression, physical inactivity, diabetes, infrequent social contact, excessive alcohol consumption, head injury, and air pollution (Livingston et al., 2020). Improving our understanding of how to prevent and treat AD/ADRD can be accelerated if we apply a systems perspective. A systems science perspective takes a complex and interdisciplinary approach to examining systems in nature, social, or any other scientific field, allowing for a deeper understanding of how individuals and populations are linked within society (Columbia Public Health, n.d.). Systems science approaches can facilitate capacity building for team-based, interdisciplinary research that engages diverse stakeholders positioned to conduct studies at multiple levels (individual, interpersonal, community, and societal), touching multiple domains of influence (biological, behavioral, physical/built environment, sociocultural environment, and health care system) (National Institute on Minority Health and Health Disparities, 2017).

The multifaceted nature of research needed to reduce the societal burden of AD/ADRD is daunting, a fact that underscores the need for methods that embrace the dynamic and nonlinear clinical characteristics of AD/ADRD morbidity as well as the imperative to identify new ways to help scientists prioritize and organize well-coordinated programs of research that synthesize and harmonize extant statistical and epidemiological evidence. Therefore, the complexities driving disparities in AD/ADRD outcomes call for innovative systems science approaches that can be used to: holistically characterize the nonlinear interdependencies between causes of AD/ADRD; identify leverageable areas in the system to inform actionable and impactful design of interventions to combat AD/ADRD; and evaluate hypothesized interventions in computer simulation environments before deployment in real-world settings.

SYSTEMS SCIENCE AND GROUP MODEL BUILDING

Systems science approaches have seen growing interest and utilization in public health, medicine, and the social sciences in recent decades (Mabry et al., 2013). This interest stems from the expanding recognition that public health problems are inherently complex and contain nonlinear interdependencies that cannot be fully characterized by linear thinking and models. Many public health research domains, including AD/ADRD, embody characteristics of a complex dynamic system as described by Sterman (2000): 1) dynamic, with trends that change over time; 2) governed by feedback, where decisions of actors alter the state of the world which in turn causes further action; 3) nonlinear, where the interaction of multiple factors during decision making produces observed effects which are not necessarily proportional to causes; 4) counterintuitive, exhibiting effects which are difficult to predict due to distant causes; and 5) policy resistant, where seemingly obvious solutions to problems fail or worsen the situation (Sterman, 2000, p. 22). While traditional research methodologies used in public health, medicine, and the social sciences no doubt continue to be useful for characterizing direct relationships and exploring narrowly focused problems, systems science approaches can expand the purview of public health research to provide more expansive insights and holistic understanding of complex public health problems (Mabry et al., 2010; Palma & Lounsbury, 2017).

Group model building (GMB) supports a participatory approach to system dynamics (SD) modeling, whereby a diverse set of stakeholders (e.g., community members, subject matter experts, government representatives) work together with modeling facilitators to build a shared understanding of the system of forces and feedbacks explaining a complex, dynamic problem. Along the way, GMB cultivates systems thinking skills among stakeholders and shapes a common agenda that prioritizes and organizes research and action to effect systems change (Estrada-Magbanua et al., 2022; Hovmand, 2013; Vennix, 1996).

There are five common steps to the SD modeling process: 1) articulation of the problem; 2) formulation of a dynamic hypothesis; 3) specification of a simulation model; 4) testing and validation of the model structure and behavior; and 5) policy design and evaluation (Sterman, 2000, p. 86). These steps do not occur as a linear sequence – rather, modeling is an ongoing, iterative process of continual questioning, testing, and refinement (Sterman, 2000, p. 87). GMB can support all steps of the SD modeling process, where GMB facilitators select and apply structured small group exercises called "scripts" that are designed to elicit the mental models of participants and build understanding of systems thinking concepts (Hovmand, 2013, pp. 23–25).

Scripts for GMB generally fall into one of four types of group activities: 1) divergent activities designed to produce an array of different ideas and interpretations; 2) convergent activities designed to cluster and categorize ideas and interpretations; 3) evaluative activities designed to rank and choose between options and ideas; and 4) presentation activities designed to educate or update participants (Hovmand, 2013, pp. 23–25). Table 7.1 gives examples of some commonly used GMB scripts (from Estrada-Magbanua et al., 2022) and a full list of scripts is available on *Scriptapedia*, a publicly available online repository of GMB scripts (Anderson et al., 2020). The information elicited from stakeholders using these scripts can then be used to support the SD modeling efforts as described above by refining the problem definition (step 1), specifying reference modes and hypothesized model structures in the form of causal loop diagrams (CLDs) and stock

TABLE 7.1 **Examples of Commonly Used GMB Scripts**

Script[a]	Description
Graphs Over Time	Participants are asked to draw multiple graphs of variables over time showing important characteristics of the issue at hand. For example, if the issue is AD/ADRD, the graph over time could be used to sketch rates of cognitive decline, number of people living with dementia, dementia caregiving costs, access and use of drugs to treat AD, over time.
Variable Elicitation	The facilitators ask participants, "What are the key variables affecting the process and outcomes of the problem at hand?" Participants write down as many problem-related variables as they can on sheets of paper and then share their list with the rest of the group. The facilitators tape the variables to a wall and cluster them according to common themes. The facilitators then prompt discussion by asking participants questions such as, "Does this resonate with you? Are there other themes you notice, or any variables you think should be moved?"
Creating a Causal Loop Diagram	The facilitators present the variables elicited from the group in the previous activity and ask the participants how the variables from the list interact and cause changes to the problem at hand. The group indicates the relationship between the variables by linking them and labeling the link with a positive (i.e., an increase in one variable will cause an increase in the other variable) or negative (i.e. an increase in one variable will cause a decrease in the other variable) polarity.
Dots	This exercise is used when there is a need to select variables, graphs, or ideas that are most important to the participant group. For example, after the variable elicitation script, participants vote on what they perceive to be the most significant variables affecting the problem at hand by placing voting dots beside the elicited variables. The facilitators then tally the dots beside each item to create a ranked list of importance.

[a]A full list of scripts may be accessed on Scriptapedia, a publicly available online repository of GMB scripts (Anderson et al., 2020).
Source: Adapted from Estrada-Magbanua et al., 2022.

and flow diagrams (SFDs) (step 2), informing specification of model parameters (step 3), strengthening model validation through stakeholder engagement and feedback elicitation (step 4), and identifying leverageable and actionable policies in light of stakeholder priorities (step 5).

At present, GMB and SD methods are underutilized in AD/ADRD research. Previous studies have used these methods to a limited extent to better understand the complex systems of factors contributing to the health of aging populations and to design and evaluate interventions to improve health outcomes of older people. Morrow-Howell et al. (2017) implemented a series of five GMB workshops engaging stakeholders with gerontology and systems science expertise to develop a qualitative SD model for productive engagement (i.e., working, volunteering, and caregiving) of older adults. This first attempt at developing a SD model for productive engagement in later life offered a new approach to advancing theory and research on productive engagement. Key insights centered on leveraging modifiable conditions within feedback loops hypothesized to drive change in productive engagement and utilization of the human capital (i.e., health status, educational attainment, and financial status) of older adults. These included: increasing capacity of organizations to engage more older adults in productive activity, which in turn promotes further organizational capacity-building (reinforcing loop 1); increasing productive engagement of older adults by organizations, leading to improved attitudes and expectations of organizations, in turn reducing age bias and promoting further engagement of older adults by organizations (reinforcing loop 2); and leveraging available human capital of older adults in productive activity, promoting further growth of human capital (as opposed to depletion due to disengagement).

Halvorsen et al. (2023) used GMB to engage participants and case managers from the Senior Community Service Employment Program (SCSEP), a federal program which provides on-the-job training to people age 55 or older having incomes below 125% of the federal poverty level and multiple barriers to employment. The purpose of this study was to gain a better understanding of how the program interacts with individual, organizational, and policy factors to influence participant well-being, as well as identify key leverage areas to further improve the program. The research team engaged GMB participants with several script activities, including: negotiating a reference mode for changes in participant well-being over the course of the SCSEP program; variable elicitation to identify factors influencing and influenced by changes in participant well-being over time; creating a CLD connecting factors between identified variables and creating feedback loops; and action ideas to identify potential intervention points to improve participant well-being. The CLD exercise revealed that the SCSEP exerts influence on multiple intersecting domains (e.g., financial, mental, social, and physical) and feedback loops influencing participant well-being, suggesting that disruptions in SCSEP participation could trigger vicious cycles which harm well-being and create barriers to further participation. The action ideas exercise elicited several respondent-driven recommendations to strengthen SCSEP which focused on preventing potential "vicious cycles" in participant well-being and eliminating barriers to participation in the program. These included reducing the "benefits cliff" by eliminating losses to safety net benefits after small increases in income, increasing opportunities for social engagement of participants, and providing individualized support to diverse participants with unique needs.

APPLYING GMB AND SD IN AD/ADRD

There is general agreement that quality of life is an important aim in research and action pursued on behalf of people with dementia and their caregivers and that individuals experiencing cognitive decline present with a complex nexus of problems and symptoms. This aim combined with the goal of supporting patient-centered (or individualized) strategies to enhance quality of life suggests that psychosocial interventions are an important first-line strategy for managing AD/ADRD morbidity and mortality (Livingston et al., 2020). Aligned with the aim of enhancing quality of life is the goal of keeping people with dementia physically healthy, as people with dementia and related conditions are more likely to have multimorbidity and frailty than others who do not, who are of similar sociodemographic background and have comparable access to care (Livingston et al., 2020).

With this focus in mind, we illustrate how GMB can be used to prioritize and organize a wide variety of research initiatives to address complex problems in AD/ADRD. We start with a conceptual framework defined by an initial reference mode (Figure 7.1) and a corresponding CLD (Figure 7.2) that is offered as a vehicle for shaping discussion and planning among AD/ADRD researchers, with the intention of prioritizing and organizing studies that examine psychosocial and behavioral influences on age-related cognitive decline. Our framework was developed by a multidisciplinary team with expertise in

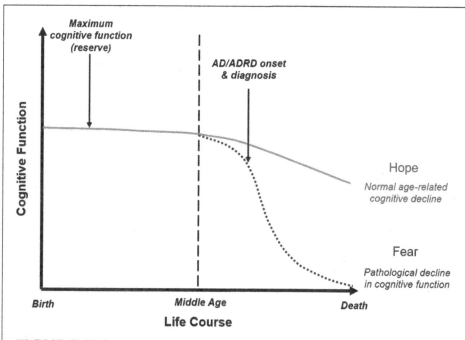

FIGURE 7.1   *Reference Mode for Dynamic Changes in Cognitive Function Over the Life Course. Source: Adapted from National Institute on Aging, 2008*

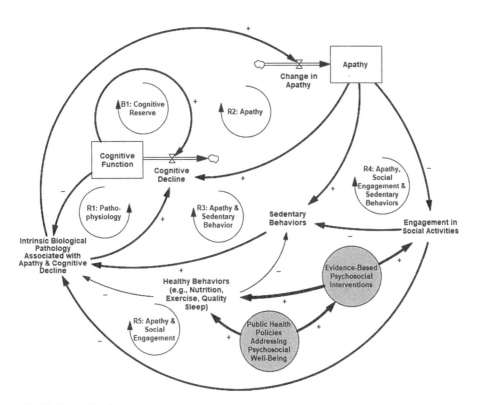

FIGURE 7.2 *CLD for Cognitive Function and Cognitive Decline in Older Adults*

psychiatry, systems science, and public health. It is intended to initiate deliberative discussion about factors and processes which may influence the rate of cognitive decline, linking expected behaviors over time to explicit reinforcing and balancing feedback mechanisms, and identifying ways to reach affected persons with evidence-based preventive strategies.

Reference modes refer to a graph, set of graphs, or other descriptive data that illustrate the developmental behavior, or trend, of a problem over time (Sterman, 2000, p. 90). A reference mode is an abstraction of the dynamic problem at hand, where quantitative data or qualitative insight can be used to inform its creation. On a graphical reference mode, the x-axis indicates the relevant time period, or time horizon, for a given problem focus. One or more variables are graphed on the y-axis, quantifying the expected mean (average) rate or level of a problem, and hypothesized desired and/or feared behavioral trajectories.

CLDs are qualitative renderings of dynamic hypotheses about the influence of one variable on another over time. Arrows linking variables in the CLD are signed positively (+) or negatively (−). If a loop has an odd number of negative (−) signs, it is said to be a balancing (or negative) loop. Balancing loops serve to stabilize the system, bringing variables into steady states (i.e., homeostasis, equilibrium). If the loop has all positive (+) signs, or an even number of negative (−) signs, it is said to be a reinforcing (or positive) loop. Reinforcing loops indicate either growth or decay over time. Reinforcing loops can also indicate the presence of a vicious cycle, where a problem becomes worse over time, often at an increasing rate (Lounsbury et al., 2014; Roberts & Anderson, 1983).

Our CLD also includes two stock-and-flow structures (see Sterman, 2000, p. 102). Stocks represent accumulations of items, actors, or information within a system (e.g., available drugs to treat AD, number of people living with dementia, perceptions of older adults' productivity). Stocks define the state of a system and drive system behavior. Flows represent activity within the system (e.g., development of drugs to treat AD, growth of the aging population and progress of dementia, change of perceptions). The action of flows changes the trajectory of a system by influencing the rate of accumulation of stocks through implicit or explicit policies. Both stocks and flows can change over time, and can represent tangible (e.g., people) or intangible (e.g., values) concepts. A stock is visually represented by a rectangular box, and a flow is depicted as an arrow with a valve in the center, coming into or out of a stock (Figure 7.2).

HYPOTHESIZED DYNAMICS OF COGNITIVE DECLINE OVER THE LIFE COURSE

Focusing on hypothesized dynamics in older adults, the reference mode defined in Figure 7.1 was adapted from the National Institute on Aging (2008) and illustrates the "hoped" and "feared" outcomes of cognitive decline over the life course. The "hoped" scenario corresponds to the normal trajectory of cognitive function (solid line), which is monotonically decreasing over the life course, albeit at a gradual rate that normally accelerates in older age. The "feared" scenario corresponds to the sudden and steep pathological decline in cognitive function in older age resulting from the development of cognitive impairment from AD/ADRD (dotted line).

With this reference mode in mind, our CLD (Figure 7.2) features cognitive function as a single stock with one outflow corresponding to the "draining" process of cognitive decline (**Cognitive Reserve Balancing Feedback Loop [B1]** with *causal path: Cognitive Function→ Cognitive Decline→ Cognitive Function*), whereby cognitive function monotonically decreases over the life course starting from a certain maximum value in early age. We then conceptualized several interacting reinforcing feedback loops that influence the rate of cognitive decline. Most of these feedback loops exert influence on the rate of cognitive decline through pathobiological processes we broadly define as, "intrinsic biological pathology." Intrinsic biological pathology refers to the underlying biological and neural changes that are associated with both apathy and cognitive decline. These include but are not limited to chronic inflammation (elevated C-reactive protein (CRP), Interleukin (IL)-6, and Tumor Necrosis Factor (TNF)-α), cerebrovascular pathology (especially in the prefrontal cortex) and decreased gray matter volume (Ceïde et al., 2022b; Eurelings et al., 2015; Grool et al., 2014; Guercio et al., 2015).

■ **Pathophysiology Reinforcing Feedback Loop [R1].** Intrinsic biological pathology contributes to an individual's rate of cognitive decline, whereby individuals who experience a greater degree of biological pathology experience faster rates of cognitive decline. Cognitive decline, by definition, leads to impairment in cognitive function (depletion of the stock of cognitive function), which in turn leads to greater acceleration of the biological pathology which contributes to even more accelerated cognitive decline. (*Causal Path: Cognitive Function→ Intrinsic Biological Pathology Associated with Apathy and Cognitive decline→ Cognitive Decline→ Cognitive Function*)

- **Apathy Reinforcing Feedback Loop [R2].** Intrinsic biological pathology can also lead to increases in apathy experienced by aging adults. A sustained apathetic state may accelerate the process of cognitive decline, causing further impairment of cognitive function which further drives pathobiological dysfunction, sustaining and increasing feelings of apathy and apathy-related changes in cognitive function. (*Causal Path: Cognitive Function→ Intrinsic Biological Pathology Associated with Apathy and Cognitive decline→ Change in Apathy→ Apathy→ Cognitive Decline→ Cognitive Function*)

- **Apathy, Social Engagement, and Sedentary Behavior Reinforcing Feedback Loops [R3 and R4].** A sustained apathetic state in older adults encourages sedentary behavior both directly [R3] and also through lack of interest in engagement in social activities [R4]. Increases in sedentary behavior contribute to further development of intrinsic biological pathology, which in turn promotes and sustains feelings of apathy. (*R3 Causal Path: Apathy→Sedentary Behaviors→ Intrinsic Biological Pathology Associated with Apathy and Cognitive decline→ Change in Apathy→ Apathy; R4 Causal Path: Apathy→Engagement in Social Activities→ Sedentary Behaviors→ Intrinsic Biological Pathology Associated with Apathy and Cognitive decline→ Change in Apathy→ Apathy*)

- **Apathy and Social Engagement Reinforcing Feedback Loop [R5].** Apathy causes aging adults to become disinterested in social activities. Lack of participation in social activities promotes cognitive decline by promoting further intrinsic biological pathology, which in turn perpetuates a state of sustained apathy and disinterest in social engagement. (*R5 Causal Path: Apathy→ Engagement in Social Activities→ Intrinsic Biological Pathology Associated with Apathy and Cognitive decline→ Change in Apathy→ Apathy*)

Our CLD emphasizes the utility of screening for apathy as an indicator of cognitive decline, as well as a potential modifiable risk factor that can be mitigated by providing opportunities for socializing and improving nutrition and sleep quality over time. A growing body of evidence indicates that apathy, a psychological syndrome characterized by lack of motivation, interest, flattening of affect, and social withdrawal (Marin et al., 1995), predicts cognitive decline including dementia (Bock et al., 2020; Ceïde et al., 2020; Clarke et al., 2010; Lanctôt et al., 2017; Rosenberg et al., 2013; van Dalen et al., 2018). Elevated biomarkers of inflammation, including CRP, TNF-α, and IL-6, have all been associated with apathy in community-dwelling older adults (Ceïde et al., 2022b; Eurelings et al., 2015). Similarly, people with cognitive impairment and apathy are more likely to have gray and white matter volume loss and increased amyloid burden (Grool et al., 2014; Marshall et al., 2013). More than just being a behavioral manifestation of underlying biology, apathy leads to social dysfunction (Groeneweg-Koolhoven et al., 2014; Lozupone et al., 2018) and decreased physical activity (Kuhlmei et al., 2013; Mulin et al., 2011; Müller et al., 2006; Valembois et al., 2015).

IDENTIFYING PRIORITIES FOR RESEARCH AND ACTION IN AD/ADRD

We propose that our conceptual framework of the dynamics of cognitive decline (Figures 7.1 and 7.2) can be readily used to foster critical dialogue by AD/ADRD researchers to help identify shared priorities that can inform the design of patient-centered psychosocial intervention studies. Aligned with Livingston et al. (2020)'s life-course model and evidence synthesis, we start with the premise that trajectories of age-related cognitive decline and/or development of AD/ADRD pathology are expected to differ by target populations or subgroups of affected people, as the rate of decline is hypothesized to be influenced by a variety of genetic, biological, social, environmental, and lifestyle factors. Our CLD helps identify areas for further discovery, dissemination, and implementation of interventions that promote healthy aging and slow the acceleration of pathological processes contributing to cognitive decline (*highlighted by gray circles in the diagram*).

For example, AD/ADRD researchers, clinicians, public health policymakers, and community AD/ADRD advocates could impact the apparent vicious cycles driving cognitive decline by promoting psychosocial well-being in individuals and at-risk populations. Evidence-based psychosocial interventions could be leveraged to promote engagement in social activities to counteract and eliminate barriers to engagement resulting from apathy. Interventions targeting and promoting healthy behaviors (e.g., sleep, nutrition, and exercise) could influence rates of cognitive decline by mitigating the impacts of intrinsic biological pathology on cognitive decline and impairment. We have also identified apathy as a critical hypothesized causal factor driving development of pathology related to cognitive decline, which could be a key target for the design and implementation of future interventions.

At this scientific juncture in AD/ADRD research, there is a particular need for community-engaged clinical trials to learn more about how to identify and engage diverse at-risk populations in evidence-based psychosocial interventions (Ceïde et al., 2016, 2022a; Kennedy & Ceïde, 2020; Livingston et al., 2020). Cultivating partnerships with community-based agencies that serve older adults will be necessary if we are to develop and bring to scale evidence-based programs. Community partners can facilitate access to settings and resources for outreach, recruitment, and retention in AD/ADRD intervention research. They can also link participants to complementary health services and to educational and vocational opportunities in the community.

SUMMARY

AD/ADRD comprise a set of mental disorders that affect a growing number of aging people but that are not yet fully understood. A complex system of biological, behavioral, and contextual factors gives rise to AD/ADRD, necessitating the use of innovative systems science approaches to fully understand complex problems in AD/ADRD research. GMB, a participatory systems science approach, is the vehicle through which systems science methods can be leveraged to expand our understanding of the nonlinear, interacting factors which give rise to AD/ADRD and establish a comprehensive, multidisciplinary, and community-centered research agenda. Using principles of GMB and SD modeling, we presented a conceptual framework for the dynamics of cognitive decline in the form of a reference mode and CLD. AD/ADRD researchers, policymakers, and community advocates can adopt or expand upon this framework as a tool for developing policy priorities, designing interventions, and fostering shared understanding of problems related to AD/ADRD through the use of GMB and other systems science techniques.

DISCUSSION QUESTIONS

1. Which feedback loop(s) describe your highest priority AD/ADRD research interest?

2. Draw one or more reference modes to illustrate the problem-focus associated with your AD/ADRD research interest. What variables did you choose to draw? What level of analysis (e.g., individual, community) and time horizon did you specify?

3. Who would you need to partner with to effectively organize and conduct your envisioned research project?

REFERENCES

Alzheimer's Association. (2022). Causes and risk factors for Alzheimer's disease. *alz.org*. Retrieved December 13, 2022, from https://www.alz.org/alzheimers-dementia/what-is-alzheimers/causes-and-risk-factors

Alzheimer's Association (2022). 2022 Alzheimer's disease facts and figures. *Alzheimer's & Dementia*, *18*(4), 700–789. https://doi.org/10.1002/alz.12638

Anderson, D. F., Calhoun, A., Hovmand, P. S., Hower, T., Rouwette, E., Steins, E., Richardson, G. P., & Rux, K. (2020). *Scriptapedia*. Retrieved December 10, 2022, from https://en.wikibooks.org/wiki/Scriptapedia

Bock, M. A., Bahorik, A., Brenowitz, W. D., & Yaffe, K. (2020). Apathy and risk of probable incident dementia among community-dwelling older adults. *Neurology*, *95*(24), e3280–e3287. https://doi.org/10.1212/WNL.0000000000010951

Ceïde, M. E., Eguchi, D., Ayers, E. I., Lounsbury, D. W., & Verghese, J. (2022b). Mediation analyses of the role of apathy on motoric cognitive outcomes. *International Journal of Environmental Research and Public Health*, *19*(12), 7376. https://doi.org/10.3390/ijerph19127376

Ceïde, M. E., Glasgow, A., Weiss, E. F., Stark, A., Kiosses, D., & Zwerling, J. L. (2022a). Feasibility of problem adaption therapy in a diverse, frail older adult population (PATH-MHS). *The American Journal of Geriatric Psychiatry: Official Journal of the American Association for Geriatric Psychiatry*, *30*(8), 917–921. https://doi.org/10.1016/j.jagp.2021.12.002

Ceïde, M. E., Nguyen, S. A., Korenblatt, J., & Kennedy, G. (2016). Beyond primary care: Integrating psychiatry into a certified home health agency to identify and treat homebound older adults with mental disorders. *Journal of Community and Medical Health Education*, *6*(479), 2161–2711.

Ceïde, M. E., Warhit, A., Ayers, E. I., Kennedy, G., & Verghese, J. (2020). Apathy and the risk of predementia syndromes in community-dwelling older adults. *The Journals of Gerontology. Series B, Psychological Sciences and Social Sciences*, *75*(7), 1443–1450. https://doi.org/10.1093/geronb/gbaa063

Clarke, D. E., Ko, J. Y., Lyketsos, C., Rebok, G. W., & Eaton, W. W. (2010). Apathy and cognitive and functional decline in community-dwelling older adults: Results from the Baltimore ECA longitudinal study. *International Psychogeriatrics*, *22*(5), 819–829. https://doi.org/10.1017/S1041610209991402

Columbia Public Health. (n.d.). Population health methods: Systems science. Available at: https://www.publichealth.columbia.edu/research/population-health-methods/systems-science

Cummings, J. L., Goldman, D. P., Simmons-Stern, N. R., & Ponton, E. (2022). The costs of developing treatments for Alzheimer's disease: A retrospective exploration. *Alzheimer's & Dementia, 18*(3), 469–477. https://doi.org/10.1002/alz.12450

Estrada-Magbanua, W. R., Huang, T. T. K., Lounsbury, D. W., Zito, P., Iftikhar, P., El-Bassel, N., Gilbert, L., Wu, E., Lee, B. Y., Mateu-Gelabert, P., & Sabounchi, N. S. (2022). *Application of group model building to implementation research: A systematic review of the public health and healthcare literature.* [Manuscript submitted for publication]. Center for Systems and Community Design and NYU-CUNY Prevention Research Center, CUNY Graduate School of Public Health and Health Policy.

Eurelings, L. S., Richard, E., Eikelenboom, P., van Gool, W. A., & Moll van Charante, E. P. (2015). Low-grade inflammation differentiates between symptoms of apathy and depression in community-dwelling older individuals. *International Psychogeriatrics, 27*(4), 639–647. https://doi.org/10.1017/S1041610214002683

Groeneweg-Koolhoven, I., de Waal, M. W., van der Weele, G. M., Gussekloo, J., & van der Mast, R. C. (2014). Quality of life in community-dwelling older persons with apathy. *The American Journal of Geriatric Psychiatry: Official Journal of the American Association for Geriatric Psychiatry, 22*(2), 186–194. https://doi.org/10.1016/j.jagp.2012.10.024

Grool, A. M., Geerlings, M. I., Sigurdsson, S., Eiriksdottir, G., Jonsson, P. V., Garcia, M. E., Siggeirsdottir, K., Harris, T. B., Sigmundsson, T., Gudnason, V., & Launer, L. J. (2014). Structural MRI correlates of apathy symptoms in older persons without dementia: AGES-Reykjavik study. *Neurology, 82*(18), 1628–1635. https://doi.org/10.1212/WNL.0000000000000378

Guercio, B. J., Donovan, N. J., Ward, A., Schultz, A., Lorius, N., Amariglio, R. E., Rentz, D. M., Johnson, K. A., Sperling, R. A., & Marshall, G. A. (2015). Apathy is associated with lower inferior temporal cortical thickness in mild cognitive impairment and normal elderly individuals. *The Journal of Neuropsychiatry and Clinical Neurosciences, 27*(1), e22–e27. https://doi.org/10.1176/appi.neuropsych.13060141

Halvorsen, C. J., Werner, K., McColloch, E., & Yulikova, O. (2023). How the senior community service employment program influences participant well-being: A participatory research approach with program recommendations. *Research on Aging, 45*(1), 77–91. https://doi.org/10.1177/01640275221098613

Hovmand, P. S. (2013). Community based system dynamics. Springer Science & Business Media.

Kennedy, G. J., & Ceïde, M. E. (2020). Bringing services to seniors rather than seniors to services: Proof of concept. *International Psychogeriatrics, 32*(4), 435–436. https://doi.org/10.1017/S1041610219001972

Kuhlmei, A., Walther, B., Becker, T., Müller, U., & Nikolaus, T. (2013). Actigraphic daytime activity is reduced in patients with cognitive impairment and apathy. *European Psychiatry: The Journal of the Association of European Psychiatrists, 28*(2), 94–97. https://doi.org/10.1016/j.eurpsy.2011.04.006

Lanctôt, K. L., Agüera-Ortiz, L., Brodaty, H., Francis, P. T., Geda, Y. E., Ismail, Z., Marshall, G. A., Mortby, M. E., Onyike, C. U., Padala, P. R., Politis, A. M., Rosenberg, P. B., Siegel, E., Sultzer, D. L., & Abraham, E. H. (2017). Apathy associated with neurocognitive disorders: Recent progress and future directions. *Alzheimer's & Dementia: The Journal of the Alzheimer's Association, 13*(1), 84–100. https://doi.org/10.1016/j.jalz.2016.05.008

Livingston, G., Huntley, J., Sommerlad, A., Ames, D., Ballard, C., Banerjee, S., Brayne, C., Burns, A., Cohen-Mansfield, J., Cooper, C., Costafreda, S. G., Dias, A., Fox, N., Gitlin, L. N., Howard, R., Kales, H. C., Kivimäki, M., Larson, E. B., Ogunniyi, A., & Mukadam, N. (2020). Dementia prevention, intervention, and care: 2020 report of the Lancet Commission. *The Lancet, 396*(10248), 413–446. https://doi.org/10.1016/S0140-6736(20)30367-6

Lounsbury, D. W., Hirsch, G. B., Vega, C., & Schwartz, C. E. (2014). Understanding social forces involved in diabetes outcomes: A systems science approach to quality-of-life research. *Quality of Life Research: An International Journal of Quality of Life Aspects of Treatment, Care and Rehabilitation, 23*(3), 959–969. https://doi.org/10.1007/s11136-013-0532-4

Lozupone, M., Panza, F., Piccininni, M., Copetti, M., Sardone, R., Imbimbo, B. P., Stella, E., D'Urso, F., Barulli, M. R., Battista, P., Grasso, A., Tortelli, R., Capozzo, R., Coppola, F., Abbrescia, D. I., Bellomo, A., Giannelli, G., Quaranta, N., Seripa, D., & Logroscino, G. (2018). Social dysfunction in older age and relationships with cognition, depression, and apathy: The GreatAGE study. *Journal of Alzheimer's Disease: JAD, 65*(3), 989–1000. https://doi.org/10.3233/JAD-180466

Mabry, P. L., Marcus, S. E., Clark, P. I., Leischow, S. J., & Méndez, D. (2010). Systems science: A revolution in public health policy research. *American Journal of Public Health, 100*(7), 1161–1163. https://doi.org/10.2105/AJPH.2010.198176

Mabry, P. L., Milstein, B., Abraido-Lanza, A. F., Livingood, W. C., & Allegrante, J. P. (2013). Opening a window on systems science research in health promotion and public health. *Health Education & Behavior: The Official Publication of the Society for Public Health Education*, *40*(1 Suppl), 5S–8S. https://doi.org/10.1177/1090198113503343

Marin, R. S., Fogel, B. S., Hawkins, J., Duffy, J., & Krupp, B. (1995). Apathy: A treatable syndrome. *The Journal of Neuropsychiatry and Clinical Neurosciences*, *7*(1), 23–30. https://doi.org/10.1176/jnp.7.1.23

Marshall, G. A., Donovan, N. J., Lorius, N., Gidicsin, C. M., Maye, J., Pepin, L. C., Becker, J. A., Amariglio, R. E., Rentz, D. M., Sperling, R. A., & Johnson, K. A. (2013). Apathy is associated with increased amyloid burden in mild cognitive impairment. *The Journal of Neuropsychiatry and Clinical Neurosciences*, *25*(4), 302–307. https://doi.org/10.1176/appi.neuropsych.12060156

Morrow-Howell, N., Halvorsen, C. J., Hovmand, P., Lee, C., & Ballard, E. (2017). Conceptualizing productive engagement in a system dynamics framework. *Innovation in Aging*, *1*(1), igx018. https://doi.org/10.1093/geroni/igx018

Mulin, E., Zeitzer, J. M., Friedman, L., Le Duff, F., Yesavage, J., Robert, P. H., & David, R. (2011). Relationship between apathy and sleep disturbance in mild and moderate Alzheimer's disease: An actigraphic study. *Journal of Alzheimer's Disease: JAD*, *25*(1), 85–91. https://doi.org/10.3233/JAD-2011-101701

Müller, U., Czymmek, J., Thöne-Otto, A., & Von Cramon, D. Y. (2006). Reduced daytime activity in patients with acquired brain damage and apathy: A study with ambulatory actigraphy. *Brain Injury*, *20*(2), 157–160. https://doi.org/10.1080/02699050500443467

National Institute on Aging (2008). Alzheimer's disease unraveling the mystery. Retrieved December 10, 2022, from https://adrccares.org/wp-content/uploads/2016/01/alzheimers_disease_unraveling_the_mystery_0.pdf

National Institute on Minority Health and Health Disparities (2017). NIMHD research framework. Retrieved December 10, 2022, from https://nimhd.nih.gov/researchFramework

Nichols, E., Steinmetz, J. D., Vollset, S. E., Fukutaki, K., Chalek, J., Abd-Allah, F., Abdoli, A., Abualhasan, A., Abu-Gharbieh, E., Akram, T. T., Hamad, H. A., Alahdab, F., Alanezi, F. M., Alipour, V., Almustanyir, S., Amu, H., Ansari, I., Arabloo, J., Ashraf, T., & Vos, T. (2022). Estimation of the global prevalence of dementia in 2019 and forecasted prevalence in 2050: An analysis for the global burden of disease study 2019. *The Lancet Public Health*, *7*(2), e105–e125. https://doi.org/10.1016/S2468-2667(21)00249-8

Palma, A., & Lounsbury, D. W. (2017). The evolution toward 21st-century science. In: A. M. El-Sayed, & S. Galea. (Eds.), Systems science and population health (p. 37), Oxford Academic.

Roberts, N., & Anderson, D. (1983). Introduction to computer simulation: A system dynamics modeling approach. Productivity Press.

Rosenberg, P. B., Mielke, M. M., Appleby, B. S., Oh, E. S., Geda, Y. E., & Lyketsos, C. G. (2013). The association of neuropsychiatric symptoms in MCI with incident dementia and Alzheimer disease. *The American Journal of Geriatric Psychiatry: Official Journal of the American Association for Geriatric Psychiatry*, *21*(7), 685–695. https://doi.org/10.1016/j.jagp.2013.01.006

Sterman, J. (2000). Business dynamics: Systems thinking and modeling for a complex world. Irwin/McGraw-Hill.

Valembois, L., Oasi, C., Pariel, S., Jarzebowski, W., Lafuente-Lafuente, C., & Belmin, J. (2015). Wrist actigraphy: A simple way to record motor activity in elderly patients with Dementia and apathy or aberrant motor behavior. *The Journal of Nutrition, Health & Aging*, *19*(7), 759–764. https://doi.org/10.1007/s12603-015-0530-z

van Dalen, J. W., Van Wanrooij, L. L., Moll van Charante, E. P., Richard, E., & van Gool, W. A. (2018). Apathy is associated with incident dementia in community-dwelling older people. *Neurology*, *90*(1), e82–e89. https://doi.org/10.1212/WNL.0000000000004767

Vennix, J. A. M. (1996). Group model building: Facilitating team learning using system dynamics. J. Wiley.

CHAPTER

8

SLEEP, AGING, AND BRAIN HEALTH

JAY M. IYER, REBECCA ROBBINS, STUART F. QUAN

LEARNING OBJECTIVES

By the end of this chapter, readers will be able to:

- Understand the normative structural components of sleep and how these components differ between younger and older individuals.
- Summarize the social and economic factors impacting sleep differences among older adults who are members of diverse racial and ethnic communities.
- Explain how sleep impacts physical, emotional, and mental health.

INTRODUCTION

Sleep is a fundamental component of human health, performance, and even survival (Buysse, 2014; Cappuccio et al., 2010; Worley, 2018). In a typical 85-year lifespan, an individual ideally will spend approximately 250,000 hours sleeping, amounting to 10,000 24-hour days (Scullin & Bliwise, 2015). Despite the importance of sleep, many adults fall short of sleep health targets, including sleep duration. According to nationally

Population Science Methods and Approaches to Aging and Alzheimer's Disease and Related Dementias Research, First Edition. Edited by Chau Trinh-Shevrin.
© 2024 John Wiley & Sons, Inc. Published 2024 by John Wiley & Sons, Inc.

representative data, approximately one in three adults in the United States do not regularly meet the recommended seven to nine hours of sleep (Y. Liu, 2016). Recent research in a nationally representative sample of United States (US) adults found that approximately two in three Americans reported not feeling restored by their sleep (Robbins, Quan et al., 2022).

As people age, moreover, marked differences emerge in the structure of their sleep and their ability to obtain sufficient sleep duration of satisfactory quality may change (Bliwise, 1993). Specifically, nocturnal total sleep duration often declines as people age, as does the quantity and quality of the "deep" stages of sleep such as slow-wave sleep (SWS) and rapid eye movement (REM) sleep (Bliwise, 1993; Ohayon et al., 2004). These changes contribute to the reasons that older adults report more sleep difficulties than younger adults (Ohayon & Vecchierini, 2005). This chapter will review the qualities of normative sleep across the lifespan. Then, it will review sleep difficulties among older adults, emotional and mental health consequences of insufficient or poor-quality sleep, the impact of sleep on physical and brain health, sleep disparities, and sleep during the novel coronavirus disease 2019 (COVID-19) pandemic among older adults.

NORMATIVE SLEEP

Normative sleep is divided into rapid eye movement (REM) and non-rapid eye movement (NREM) sleep (Kryger et al., 2017) (Figure 8.1). NREM sleep is further divided into three sleep stages, namely N1, N2, and N3 (Berry et al.).

REM sleep is characterized by decreased electroencephalogram (EEG) amplitude and episodic rapid eye movement. As one begins to fall asleep, there is a transition from wakefulness to light NREM (N1) sleep (Kryger et al., 2017). NREM sleep deepens to slow-wave sleep and eventually REM sleep occurs. The entire NREM-REM cycle can vary in length from 90 to 120 minutes and is repeated four to five times per night. N1 is the transition stage, representing 2–5% of total sleep time (TST), while N2 represents 45–55%. N3, also termed slow-wave sleep (SWS) because of its characteristic slower and higher amplitude waveforms, represents 10–20% of total sleep, and REM sleep occupies 20–25% of a typical night (Kryger et al., 2017). Extremes of sleep duration with varying amounts of time spent in each sleep stage influence risk of adverse health outcomes, such as risk of infectious and inflammatory disease (Dew et al., 2003; Irwin, 2015; Kripke et al., 2002; Mallon et al., 2002; Vgontzas et al., 2013). Sleep disorders may also cause improper time spent in each sleep stage, with 25% of the population reporting insomnia complaints, many of which represent deviations from normative sleep staging (LeBlanc et al., 2009).

Unfortunately, insufficient sleep (less than the recommended seven to nine hours per night) is becoming increasingly prevalent in the population (Matricciani et al., 2012). Insufficient sleep is associated with many adverse health outcomes, ranging from sleep disorders to neurologic and cardiovascular disease (Anic et al., 2010; Grandner et al., 2010; Knutson, 2010). Research documents that 34.8% of people overall attain less than the "acceptable sleep duration," (< 7 hours per night), and one in four people sleeps less than their age-specific recommendation (Kocevska et al., 2021; Y. Liu, 2016). The most striking group is teenagers, with 51.5% reporting a TST of less than the recommended eight to ten hours per night and 18% reporting daytime sleepiness (Kocevska et al., 2021). In adults,

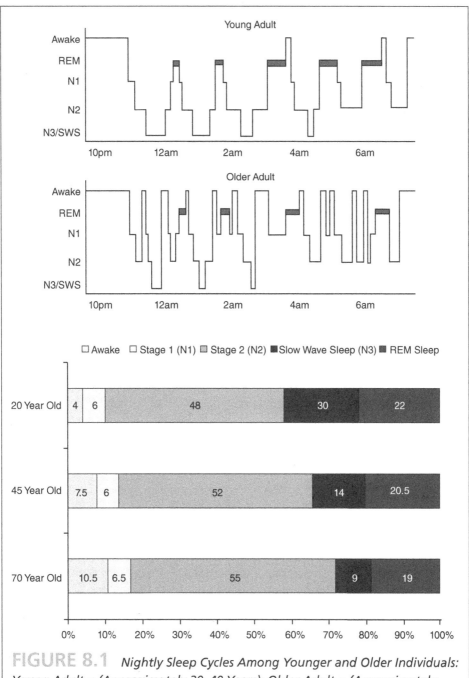

FIGURE 8.1 *Nightly Sleep Cycles Among Younger and Older Individuals: Young Adult = (Approximately 20–40 Years); Older Adult = (Approximately 65–80 Years); REM = Rapid Eye Movement Sleep; N1 = Stage One, N2 = Stage 2, N3/ SWS = Slow-wave Sleep*

however, insomnia symptoms are more common than short sleep duration (Kocevska et al., 2021). Further, women older than 41 years of age reported sleeping shorter and less efficiently than men of the same age (Kocevska et al., 2021).

SLEEP CHANGES OVER THE LIFESPAN

In humans, sleep patterns change throughout the aging process, which is caused by a variety of different factors (D. Foley et al., 2004). Variability in bedtimes and waketimes, shorter nighttime sleep duration, increased number of naps during the day, more nighttime awakenings and time spent awake, and decreased SWS are all sleep characteristics that begin to emerge as one ages (Ohayon et al., 2004). These changes begin to appear during early adulthood, as sleep efficiency remains relatively unchanged from childhood to adolescence but decreases in adulthood (Ohayon et al., 2004).

Those over age 60 years commonly experience reduced ability to maintain sleep, fall asleep, and fall back to sleep after nighttime awakenings (Floyd et al., 2000; Ohayon et al., 2004). Furthermore, older adults report lower sleep quality than do younger adults, which partially may be attributed to a reduction in SWS and an increase in daytime napping (Foley et al., 1999; Furihata et al., 2017; Luo et al., 2013; Pótári et al., 2017; Vitiello et al., 2004). However, the causes of sleep changes due to aging are multifactorial, and can be divided into biological, social, and cultural factors. Age-related changes in neuroendocrine functions correlate with changes in sleep quantity and quality (Kryger et al., 2017). Growth hormone (GH) secretion decreases quickly after young adulthood and middle age, then more slowly, and is associated with less SWS (Copinschi & Caufriez, 2013; Van Cauter et al., 2000; van Coevorden et al., 1991). Further, circadian system and sleep-related hormone secretion are less robust in normal aging, potentially causing lowered ability for an individual to obtain a healthy amount of sleep (Mattis & Sehgal, 2016). Social causes of sleep changes and negative effects on sleep in older adults include environment changes, social engagement, and overall lifestyle (Vaughan & Bliwise, 2018). The aforementioned are examples of the multifactorial nature of changes in sleep characteristics in aging individuals.

SLEEP DIFFICULTIES AMONG OLDER ADULTS

Insomnia

The risk for developing sleep disorders increases with age (Miner & Kryger, 2017). The proportion of older adults as a percentage of the overall US population continues to grow over time due to increased life expectancy, but there is a lack of emphasis placed on sleep disorders in relation to well-being among older people (Gulia & Kumar, 2018). Insomnia, defined as a sleep disorder characterized by the symptoms of having trouble falling and/or staying asleep in conjunction with an impairment in daytime functioning, is one of the most common sleep disorders in older people (Rosenberg & Van Hout, 2014). This is consistent with an overall general dissatisfaction with sleep quantity or quality associated with sleep initiation and maintenance among older adults (Widiger et al., 2013).

An increased prevalence of insomnia symptoms in older individuals is a consistent finding of almost every epidemiologic study that has been conducted. For example, in one large-scale epidemiological study, 23% to 34% of individuals older than 65 complained of symptoms that were consistent with a clinical diagnosis of insomnia, with over 50% reporting difficulties sleeping (Ebben, 2021; Foley et al., 1995). Relatedly, napping was reported in approximately 25% of older adults, which may be a reflection of sleep difficulties (Ebben, 2021; Foley et al., 1995). However, after controlling for mental and medical health conditions, the prevalence of insomnia in older adults was similar to younger populations (Foley et al., 1995). This suggests that the increased prevalence of insomnia in older adults, in large part, may be related to issues inherent to the aging process itself, such as declines in physical and mental health. Nevertheless, as demonstrated in recent prospective studies, insomnia symptoms are associated with worse cognitive function (Etholén et al., 2022; Li et al., 2018) and, in at least one additional study conducted across eight years, sleep difficulties were associated with incident dementia and all-cause mortality among older adults (Robbins et al., 2019).

Untreated insomnia may have serious negative impacts on overall health and well-being, particularly among older people. For example, untreated and hypnotic-treated insomnia are risk factors for falls among older individuals (Avidan et al., 2005; Gureje et al., 2009; Stone et al., 2008). Furthermore, difficulty initiating and maintaining sleep was associated with a moderate increase in acute myocardial infarction risk in a cohort of both younger and older adults in Norway followed over 11.4 years (Laugsand et al., 2011). Among older people in Japan, markers of carotid vascular disease were found to be elevated in participants with insomnia and those that slept less than five hours per night (Nakazaki et al., 2012). Persistent insomnia may be a risk factor for premature death (Parthasarathy et al., 2015). Treatment of adult patients, including older individuals, who have chronic insomnia may include pharmacotherapy, cognitive behavioral therapy (CBT), or a combination of both. However, the recommended intervention for insomnia in older people is cognitive behavioral therapy for insomnia (CBT-i). CBT-i is a program that combines elimination of thoughts and behaviors that may be preventing an individual from sleeping and maintaining sleep with behavioral interventions to facilitate sleep (Morgenthaler et al., 2006). CBT-i is preferred over pharmacotherapy because its favorable effect on insomnia is more enduring than pharmacological intervention. (Kay-Stacey & Attarian, 2016; Sateia et al., 2017; Schroeck et al., 2016). Other psychological/behavioral therapies have been used successfully to treat older individuals with insomnia, as well (Abad & Guilleminault, 2018; Black et al., 2015; Irwin, 2015; Lovato et al., 2014; Morgan et al., 2012; Morin et al., 1999; Omvik et al., 2008; Rybarczyk et al., 2005; Sivertsen et al., 2006).

Restless Legs Syndrome

Another common sleep disorder among older people is Restless Legs Syndrome (RLS), which is characterized by abnormal burning, tingling, and numbness in the legs typically occurring in the evening at bedtime (Milligan & Chesson, 2002). RLS is estimated to affect between 10 and 35% of individuals over 65 years of age, and its symptoms result in the individual moving their legs to temporarily relieve the abnormal sensations (Milligan & Chesson, 2002). Due to the nature of uncontrollable movement to relieve symptoms, many people affected by this condition develop insomnia (Milligan & Chesson, 2002). In most cases, RLS appears to be related to dysfunction of dopamine metabolism in the brain. Therefore, symptoms of RLS are frequently managed with dopaminergic therapy, such as levodopa-carbidopa, and dopamine-receptor agonists including pramipexole and ropinirole (Milligan & Chesson, 2002). However, a deficit in brain iron is associated with RLS in some individuals and iron supplementation often decreases the severity of RLS (Trotti & Becker, 2019).

Sleep Apnea

Along with insomnia and RLS, sleep apnea – particularly, obstructive sleep apnea (OSA) – is highly prevalent in older adults and may accelerate signs of physical and mental decline associated with aging (Benca & Teodorescu, 2019; Gaspar et al., 2017). The estimated prevalence rates of OSA in 50–70 year-old men and women are 17.4% and 9.1%, respectively (Peppard et al., 2013). OSA is characterized by repetitive episodes of complete (apnea) or partial obstruction (hypopnea) of the upper airway, resulting in intermittent episodes of hypoxia and sleep fragmentation. The latter commonly results in daytime sleepiness, one of the cardinal symptoms of the disorder. Older adults with OSA often have comorbid respiratory and cardiovascular disorders (Okuro & Morimoto, 2014). It has been hypothesized that OSA can induce cellular and molecular changes that define aging (Gaspar et al., 2017). In addition to accelerating and potentially causing the onset of aging and aging-related symptoms, OSA can impair sleep-dependent memory consolidation in the absence of neurological changes (Pace-Schott & Spencer, 2015).

Increasing evidence suggests a correlation between sleep patterns reported in Alzheimer's Disease (AD) and OSA, such as EEG slowing (Mullins et al., 2020). Continuous positive airway pressure (CPAP) therapy, the most common treatment for OSA, often ameliorates symptoms and may reverse metabolic, biochemical, inflammatory, and physiologic changes induced by OSA but there is a lack of longitudinal studies in this area (Mullins et al., 2020). OSA can also cause symptoms similar to patients with AD, such as lower attention and physical response times, as well as memory impairments (Berkley, 2021). In fact, it has been shown that OSA may be a common risk factor for AD and play a role in the latter's development. (Bombois et al., 2010).

Short Sleep Duration

In contrast to sleep disorders such as insomnia and sleep apnea, overall total sleep time during a 24-hour period does not change in old- versus middle-aged healthy adults without sleep symptoms. However, nocturnal sleep duration is reduced and may be interpreted by some older adults as being abnormal.

Social factors also influence sleep duration in older adults, as shown by a study using the 2014–2018 National Health Interview Survey that analyzed heterosexual married adults aged 50–84 (Sheehan & Iida, 2021). Study participants reported typical sleep duration in a 24-hour period and the study found that older adults married to spouses with college or more education had a significantly lower risk of short sleep than those whose spouses had some college, high school, or less than high school education (Sheehan & Iida, 2021). Further, older adults who are married reported a longer sleep duration than those unmarried (Chen et al., 2015).

Lastly, there are mixed findings in the literature related to the associations between sleep duration and mortality. One study analyzed sleep disturbance and deficiency across five years in a nationally representative sample of older adults in the United States containing 2,812 individuals and showed that poor/very poor sleep quality and extremely short sleep duration (<6 hours) were both associated with all-cause mortality (Robbins et al., 2021). On the other hand, sleep duration may not have an association with mortality among older adults. In a Swedish prospective cohort study in which 43,863 individuals were followed through record linkages for 13 years (Åkerstedt et al., 2017), sleep duration was self-reported and grouped into four categories (<5, 6, 7, and >8 hours). Among individuals less than 65 years of age, short (<5 h) and long (>8 h) sleep duration showed a significant relationship with mortality (Åkerstedt et al., 2017). Among individuals greater than 65 years old, no relationships between sleep duration and mortality were observed. The greatest effect of short and long sleep duration on mortality was highest among young adults and decreased as aging progressed (Åkerstedt et al., 2017).

Physical and Brain Health Effects

Emerging data suggest that sleep duration and quality in older adults may have profound impacts on physical and brain health. One cross-sectional study involving 392 non-institutionalized adults aged over 65 years assessed sleep quality using the Pittsburgh Sleep Quality Index (PSQI). Poor sleep quality (PSQI ≥10) was associated with muscle weakness, frailty, and poor physical performance (Arias-Fernández et al., 2021). Participants with poor sleep quality (PSQI ≥ 10) also were more likely to have functional limitations. Lower Extremity Functional Impairment was associated with poor sleep efficiency, while subjective poor sleep quality and daytime dysfunction were linked to muscle weakness (Arias-Fernández et al., 2021).

Another observational study including 1,781 participants over 65 years of age assessed relationships among self-reported sleep duration and quality and clinically evaluated body mass index and waist circumference (Mamalaki et al., 2019). Sleep duration was inversely related to waist circumference only in women after adjusting for age, gender, education, and level of physical activity (Mamalaki et al., 2019). This finding suggests that poor sleep may be associated with adverse weight effects in older women but not men (Mamalaki et al., 2019). Further relationships between sleep duration and physical function in older individuals were elucidated by a cross-sectional study which evaluated the sleep duration of people aged 60 years and older using accelerometers. To assess physical function, researchers measured participants' grip strength, balance, lower body strength, mobility, and gait speed (Huang et al., 2021). A positive association of sleep duration with grip strength was found after adjusting for potential covariates but no significant associations were observed between sleep duration and other physical function outcomes (Huang et al., 2021). This finding suggests that adequate sleep duration may be important in maintaining muscle strength in older adults (Huang et al., 2021).

Researchers have also uncovered potential negative effects of sleep difficulties on brain and cognitive health. In a cross-sectional study including 3,086 older adults aged 60 years or older, replacing sedentary activities with moderate-vigorous physical activity was associated with more favorable cognitive function among older adults sleeping less than 7 hours a night (Wei et al., 2021). Furthermore, replacing excessive sleep with sedentary or physical activities was also associated with favorable cognition (Wei et al., 2021). This study showed that it is possible to remediate the negative cognitive impacts of sleeping difficulties in older adults with physical exercise. Furthermore, in a meta-analysis of observational studies that included 35 independent samples assessing associations between sleep duration and cognitive performance, it was found that self-reported "extreme" sleep duration is a major risk factor for cognitive aging (Lo et al., 2016).

EMOTIONAL AND MENTAL HEALTH CONSEQUENCES OF INSUFFICIENT SLEEP

Emotional Consequences of Insufficient Sleep and Sleep Difficulties

Sleep plays a critical role in supporting emotional and mental health. More specifically, sleep duration is fundamental to proper emotional regulation and sleep deprivation has a significant negative effect on emotional processing (Deliens et al., 2014; Shen et al., 2018). This is partially due to the fact that emotional processing may be conducted during deep REM sleep (Tempesta et al., 2018). Using structural equation modeling, one study found that ensuring proper sleep duration may promote more positive emotions and reduce mood fluctuations (Shen et al., 2018). Furthermore, a study that analyzed the association between sleep quality and emotions using the PSQI found that there is a different day and night expression of emotions between individuals marked as "good sleepers" and those identified as "poor sleepers." The "good sleeper" group had a shift in emotionality from positive to negative between wakefulness and dreams, respectively (Conte et al., 2021). Conversely, "poor sleepers" showed an evenly distributed emotionality between wakefulness and dreaming. These data suggest that the expression of emotions between groups is directly dependent upon the degree to which sleep-related processes have disrupted emotional regulation (Conte et al., 2021). The fact that emotional processing in the brain may be sleep-dependent could lead to new investigations to fully elucidate any potential causal relationship between poor sleep and the onset of these disorders (Walker, 2009). Additionally, it is still unknown which specific components of emotions are dependent on sleep regulation (Palmer & Alfano, 2017).

Mental Health Consequences of Insufficient Sleep and Sleep Difficulties

Insufficient sleep and sleep difficulties may be associated with adverse mental health outcomes. A meta-analysis that analyzed randomized controlled trials (RCTs) assessing the association between sleep duration and mental health concluded that short sleep duration is causally related to mental health difficulties (Scott et al., 2021). One large cross-sectional study conducted in the United Kingdom suggested associations between nighttime sleep duration and mental health problems as well as psychological distress, while a US-based cross-sectional study of college students suggested a positive association between sleep and mental health (Hepsomali & Groeger, 2021; Milojevich & Lukowski, 2016). This association is further supported by a cross-sectional study that included 273,695 adults, showing that participants who averaged six hours of sleep or less were 2.5 times more likely to experience mental distress than those who slept more than six hours (Blackwelder et al., 2021). Another study using multivariable logistic regression also observed that insufficient sleep (< 7 hours) increased risk for depression among 25,962 US adults (Dong et al., 2022). Further, a meta-analysis analyzing polysomnographic studies – i.e., those that record brain waves, blood oxygen levels, heart rate, and breathing in order to diagnose sleep disorders

(Markun & Sampat, 2020) – showed that sleep continuity problems are observed in most mental disorders, such as autism, schizophrenia, and other disorders (Baglioni et al., 2016). At least one cross-sectional study has also shown that poor sleep quality may be associated with depression, anxiety, and stress – conditions that have been identified as risk factors for additional mental disorders (Al-Khani et al., 2019).

Fortunately, there are treatments that have proven effective in managing insufficient sleep and sleep difficulties and, in turn, reducing the risk of negative impacts on emotional and brain health. In RCTs, CBT-i and positive mood strategies (CBT-i+) generated a greater reduction in insomnia and depression severity compared to a psychoeducation control group (PCG) (Sadler et al., 2018). Furthermore, moderate-level physical activity positively affects aspects of sleep in healthy older adults, particularly when carried out as part of organized exercise programs (Vanderlinden et al., 2020).

SLEEP AND BRAIN HEALTH

Impact of Sleep on Brain Health

One of the most important functions of sleep is to support normal brain health (Murillo-Rodriguez et al., 2012). Biochemically, sleep maintains the physiological health of the human brain through the maintenance of fluid and neuronal activity, enabling synaptic plasticity (Frank, 2015; Lewis, 2021). This process allows for specific brain mechanisms to regulate sleep/wake cycles, coordinating them with dynamic environmental and behavioral demands (Schneider, 2020). Sleep also serves a neuroprotective purpose, potentially slowing the progression of neurodegenerative disorders (Eugene & Masiak, 2015). A key laboratory study showed that fluxes of interstitial fluid increase the rate of beta-amyloid clearance during sleep, suggesting a protective benefit of sleep against the onset and progression of neurodegenerative disorders (Xie et al., 2013). In parallel, in the largest neuroimaging study conducted to date, researchers found that individuals who slept six to eight hours a night had more gray matter volume in 46 of 139 brain regions as compared to those who reported sleeping less than six hours or greater than eight hours per night (Tai et al., 2022). This finding suggests that the former group had less neurodegeneration than the latter.

While many possible explanations for the mechanisms through which sleep supports brain health have been proposed, two key hypotheses merit discussion here. The metabolic waste hypothesis suggests that sleep eliminates toxins (e.g., reactive oxygen species) that accumulate in the brain as a result of metabolic activity. In contrast, the restorative hypothesis posits that sleep allows for the body to repair and replete cellular components that are depleted during the daytime, thereby maintaining brain metabolic activity (Frank & Heller, 2019). Irrespective of which hypothesis is eventually proven, sleep is a critical component of maintaining healthy brain chemistry.

Sleep and Aging-Related Brain Disorders

Dementia In general, dementia is an "acquired loss of cognition" that affects a host of functional domains, including day-to-day and social activities (Arvanitakis et al., 2019). The most common form of dementia is AD (Arvanitakis et al., 2019). Other forms of dementia include stroke, which leads to vascular dementia; protein accumulation (Lewy Bodies); Parkinson's disease (PD); frontotemporal dementia; and mixed dementia resulting from a combination of AD and vascular dementia (Alzheimer's Association). A meta-analysis published in 2018 analyzed 12,926 papers to assess overall sleep disturbances and their subtypes as potential predictors of dementia (Shi et al., 2018). Out of these papers, there were 18 longitudinal studies that included over 240,000 subjects at baseline and over 25,000 cases of dementia (Shi et al., 2018). The landmark study separated the analysis of the papers into two groups: (1) subjects who reported sleep disturbances, and (2) subjects who did not report sleep disturbances (Shi et al., 2018). Comparing these two groups, subjects who reported sleep disturbances had a higher risk of dementia than subjects who did not report sleep disturbances, suggesting that sleep disturbances are an informative predictor of incident dementia (Shi et al., 2018).

Alzheimer's Disease AD is neurological disorder that is characterized by the degeneration and eventual death of neurons in the brain, thereby erasing memories and cognitive ability (Breijyeh & Karaman, 2020). It is the main cause of dementia, causing a decline in cognitive function and a disruption in routine daily activities (Breijyeh & Karaman, 2020). AD has been shown to be associated with sleep-related disorders. In a meta-analysis of 24 studies, patients with AD presented with significant reductions in total sleep time, sleep efficiency, and overall percentage of SWS and REM (Zhang et al., 2022). Further, studies have found a conclusive link between sleep quality and progression of AD, enabling researchers to use changes in the proportions of sleep stages to distinguish AD patients from controls with high accuracy (Liguori et al., 2020; S. Liu et al., 2020). One of the hallmarks of sleep in a patient with AD is the alteration of K-complex (KC) density, a wave form that is identified on EEG which occurs during N2 NREM sleep, along with sleep spindles, bursts of neural activity during N2, which are also seen in this stage (Gandhi & Emmady, 2022; Reda et al., 2017). Indeed, at least one study has shown that the alteration of KC density has only been shown in the "mature" phases of AD, and is linked to deterioration in cognitive function (Reda et al., 2017). Yet more research is needed to clarify this association. At least one other team has shown that AD-related changes in spindle density are also related to cognitive decline and have an early onset in AD pathology (Gorgoni et al., 2016).

Researchers have also examined the cause and effect of poor sleep and sleep disorders on the onset and progression of AD. For example, evidence from a study performed on OSA and AD patients concluded that sleep disruption may induce the dysregulation of beta-amyloid metabolism, suggesting that OSA may start the processes to induce AD (Liguori et al., 2019). To further investigate the cause of poor sleep in AD, at least one research team has looked at single-nucleotide polymorphisms and found that interleukin-1β promoter enhances the risk of sleep disturbances in AD (Yin et al., 2016). Hallmarks of aging-related sleep changes have been seen in patients with AD, including increased sleep propensity during the daytime and daytime sleepiness – the latter being associated with the elevation of serum TNF-α concentrations, a marker of acute inflammation. It has also been shown that there is an increase in theta activity in patients with AD to maintain memory performance, which is indicative of a "compensatory mechanism" to alleviate the stress of AD on the body and memory (Hot et al., 2011).

Parkinson's Disease Poor sleep and sleep disorders throughout adulthood are associated with increased risk for developing PD, a neurological disorder characterized by the loss of dopaminergic neurons in the substantia nigra (Poewe et al., 2017). In a prospective population-based study, it was found that worsening sleep quality and shortened sleep duration were associated with greater PD risk in the subsequent six years (Lysen et al., 2019). The study concluded that lower sleep quality and duration are indicative of the prodromal phase of PD (Lysen et al., 2019). While poor sleep confers a risk for developing PD and PD-like symptoms, patients with PD also report sleep difficulties.

General fatigue is a frequent and independent nonmotor symptom in PD which appears early and persists throughout disease progression (Siciliano et al., 2018). Even so, PD patients have poor sleep quality and quantity, as reported by polysomnographic studies (Zhang et al., 2020). Furthermore, sleep disorders, including REM Sleep Behavior Disorder (RBD), OSA, and RLS play a significant role in accelerating PD progression. These sleep disorders in patients with PD are associated with global cognitive dysfunction, and increased risk of long-term cognitive decline (Maggi et al., 2021). For example, there was an overall higher score on the Unified Parkinson's Disease Rating Scale (UPDRS III) in patients with OSA when compared to those without OSA (Elfil et al., 2021).

DISPARITIES IN SLEEP HEALTH

The relationship between sleep and aging is highly dependent on a variety of social, cultural, and socioeconomic factors that are collectively referred to as the social determinants of health (SDOH), although research is generally limited with respect to older racial and ethnic groups (Robbins et al., 2019). As discussed more extensively in Chapter 6, SDOH are the general conditions in which an individual lives, works, and ages, and in turn impact their health and quality of life. SDOH impact sleep patterns and sleep quality. Racism, historical divestment in low-income and racial and ethnic minoritized communities, and limited access to high-quality health care are all examples of SDOH that contribute to poorer sleep quality (Grandner, 2017). Importantly, emerging research suggests that sleep mediates the link between discrimination and mental health in racial and ethnic minoritized groups, highlighting the importance of considering the impact of race and environmental factors in investigations of sleep and mental health (Yip & Cheon, 2020).

People who are members of racial and ethnic minoritized populations are more likely to obtain less than the recommended amount of sleep (< 7 hours) than non-Hispanic White (White) people, with the exception of Hispanic (Latine) people not born in the United States (Jackson et al., 2020; Johnson et al., 2019). Asian American people have reported higher than normal sleepiness and commonly sleep fewer than seven hours in a typical day (Carnethon et al., 2016; Whinnery et al., 2014). In New York City, Asian American yellow taxi drivers reported insufficient sleep on work nights and approximately 37% of those surveyed were at high risk for developing OSA (Robbins, Trinh-Shevrin et al., 2022). Among Latine people, one of fastest growing and most diverse ethnic groups in the United States, significant disparities in sleep duration and sleep problems have been reported in comparison to other racial and ethnic groups. Variation among Latine subgroups was also pronounced (Baldwin et al., 2010). Among Latine people, differences in sleep patterns have also been documented between US and foreign-born individuals. One study found that foreign-born Latine individuals were more likely to obtain the recommended amount of sleep as compared to White people, a nuance that contrasts directly with research that has shown race/ethnicity to be a predictor of short sleep duration and suggests that immigration-related factors may be important to explore in relation to sleep health among racial and ethnic minoritized populations (Jackson et al., 2020; Johnson et al., 2019). Furthermore, research using data from the multicenter Sleep Heart Health study demonstrated that Latine people overall have a higher probability of snoring as compared to White people, a key marker of OSA that suggests a higher prevalence of sleep disordered breathing and poorer sleep quality (Baldwin et al., 2010).

Research among other racial and ethnic groups, including non-Hispanic Black (Black), American Indian/Alaskan Native (AI/AN), and Native Hawaiian/Pacific Islander (NH/PI) older people, is limited. However, one study conducted among older Black adults with disabilities found that measures of long sleep and wake after sleep onset (WASO) are associated with poor physical function (Okoye et al., 2021). Another study which profiled 398 economically disadvantaged Black older adults in Los Angeles found that higher financial difficulty was associated with increased frequency and risk of developing clinical insomnia (Bazargan et al., 2019). This study highlights the critical need to address sleep in economically disadvantaged areas in order to alleviate social and health challenges among these populations (Bazargan et al., 2019). Multiple surveys and epidemiological studies also have noted frequent insufficient sleep in adults who identify as AI/AN by the metrics of sleeping less than seven hours per night, or reporting 14 or more days out of 30 in which an individual did not sleep an adequate amount (Chapman et al., 2013; Ehlers et al., 2017).

SLEEP AMONG OLDER ADULTS AMIDST COVID-19

The COVID-19 pandemic has had a profound impact on the daily lives of all Americans, affecting work and school schedules and impacting almost every sector of the economy (Giuntella et al., 2021). Changes in lifestyles due to the pandemic have been associated with increased sleep duration and later sleep timing due to individuals not having to commute to work, but this may change once policies shift (Yuan et al., 2022). Indeed, COVID-19 has been associated with a later waking time and more daytime napping, particularly among older adults, which has been shown to contribute to the onset of sleep disorders (Gupta et al., 2020). These lifestyle changes have led to increased prevalence of sleep problems during the pandemic, now affecting roughly 40% of the general population (Jahrami et al., 2021). Studies have shown that these sleeping problems are also associated with higher psychological distress (Alimoradi et al., 2021). In contrast to older adults, COVID-19 has had a seemingly beneficial impact on the sleep patterns of young adults, enabling young adults to increase sleep duration and reduce daytime sleepiness (Ramos Socarras et al., 2021). However, the shift to increased sleep duration and a subsequent reduction once policies shift present broader adverse effects as shown by detrimental impacts to student well-being (Ellakany et al., 2022).

SUMMARY

Sleep is a cornerstone of human health, functioning, and well-being. Sleep changes across the lifespan, such that older adults can face challenges when it comes to sleep. Moreover, health disparities in sleep outcomes demonstrate that members of underserved communities and racial and ethnic minoritized communities are at greater risk for insufficient sleep, among other poor sleep health indicators.

DISCUSSION QUESTIONS

1. What are some of the challenges in further understanding of the impact of social and racial and ethnic disparities on sleep health in an aging population?

2. What additional evidence is needed to better define the role of disordered sleep in the development of AD?

3. What are the mechanisms through which extremes of sleep duration are associated with detrimental mental and physical health effects in older adults?

REFERENCES

Abad, V. C., & Guilleminault, C. (2018). Insomnia in elderly patients: Recommendations for pharmacological management. *Drugs & Aging*, *35*(9), 791–817. https://doi.org/10.1007/s40266-018-0569-8

Kay-Stacey, M., & Attarian, H. (2016). Advances in the management of chronic insomnia. BMJ (*Clinical Research Ed.*), 354, i2123. https://doi.org/10.1136/bmj.i2123

Åkerstedt, T., Ghilotti, F., Grotta, A., Bellavia, A., Lagerros, Y. T., & Bellocco, R. (2017). Sleep duration, mortality and the influence of age. *European Journal of Epidemiology*, *32*(10), 881–891. https://doi.org/10.1007/s10654-017-0297-0

Alimoradi, Z., Broström, A., Tsang, H. W. H., Griffiths, M. D., Haghayegh, S., Ohayon, M. M., Lin, C.Y., & Pakpour, A. H. (2021). Sleep problems during COVID-19 pandemic and its' association to psychological distress: A systematic review and meta-analysis. *EClinicalMedicine*, *36*, 100916. https://doi.org/10.1016/j.eclinm.2021.100916

Al-Khani, A. M., Sarhandi, M. I., Zaghloul, M. S., Ewid, M., & Saquib, N. (2019). A cross-sectional survey on sleep quality, mental health, and academic performance among medical students in Saudi Arabia. *BMC Research Notes*, *12*(1), 665. https://doi.org/10.1186/s13104-019-4713-2

Anic, G. M., Titus-Ernstoff, L., Newcomb, P. A., Trentham-Dietz, A., & Egan, K. M. (2010). Sleep duration and obesity in a population-based study. *Sleep Medicine*, *11*(5), 447–451. https://doi.org/10.1016/j.sleep.2009.11.013

Arias-Fernández, L., Smith-Plaza, A. M., Barrera-Castillo, M., Prado-Suárez, J., Lopez-Garcia, E., Rodríguez-Artalejo, F., & Lana, A. (2021). Sleep patterns and physical function in older adults attending primary health care. *Family Practice*, *38*(2), 147–153. https://doi.org/10.1093/fampra/cmaa085

Arvanitakis, Z., Shah, R. C., & Bennett, D. A. (2019). Diagnosis and management of Dementia: A review. *JAMA*, *322*(16), 1589–1599. https://doi.org/10.1001/jama.2019.4782

Avidan, A. Y., Fries, B. E., James, M. L., Szafara, K. L., Wright, G. T., & Chervin, R. D. (2005). Insomnia and hypnotic use, recorded in the minimum data set, as predictors of falls and hip fractures in Michigan nursing homes. *Journal of the American Geriatrics Society*, *53*(6), 955–962. https://doi.org/10.1111/j.1532-5415.2005.53304.x

Baglioni, C., Nanovska, S., Regen, W., Spiegelhalder, K., Feige, B., Nissen, C., Reynolds, C. F., & Riemann, D. (2016). Sleep and mental disorders: A meta-analysis of polysomnographic research. *Psychological Bulletin*, *142*(9), 969–990. https://doi.org/10.1037/bul0000053

Baldwin, C., Reynaga-Ornelas, L., Caudillo-Cisneros, C., Márquez-Gamiño, S., & Quan, S. (2010). Overview of sleep disorders among Latinos in the United States. *Hispanic Health Care International, 8.* https://doi.org/10.1891/1540-4153.8.4.180

Bazargan, M., Mian, N., Cobb, S., Vargas, R., & Assari, S. (2019). Insomnia symptoms among African-American older adults in economically disadvantaged areas of South Los Angeles. *Brain Sciences, 9*(11), 306. https://doi.org/10.3390/brainsci9110306

Benca, R. M., & Teodorescu, M. (2019). Sleep physiology and disorders in aging and dementia. *Handbook of Clinical Neurology, 167,* 477–493. https://doi.org/10.1016/B978-0-12-804766-8.00026-1

Berkley, A. S. (2021). Sleep, aging, and daily functioning. *The Nursing Clinics of North America, 56*(2), 287–298. https://doi.org/10.1016/j.cnur.2021.02.007

Black, D. S., O'Reilly, G. A., Olmstead, R., Breen, E. C., & Irwin, M. R. (2015). Mindfulness meditation and improvement in sleep quality and daytime impairment among older adults with sleep disturbances: A randomized clinical trial. *JAMA Internal Medicine, 175*(4), 494–501. https://doi.org/10.1001/jamainternmed.2014.8081

Blackwelder, A., Hoskins, M., & Huber, L. (2021). Effect of inadequate sleep on frequent mental distress. *Preventing Chronic Disease, 18,* E61. https://doi.org/10.5888/pcd18.200573

Bliwise, D. L. (1993). Sleep in normal aging and dementia. *Sleep, 16*(1), 40–81. https://doi.org/10.1093/sleep/16.1.40

Bombois, S., Derambure, P., Pasquier, F., & Monaca, C. (2010). Sleep disorders in aging and dementia. *The Journal of Nutrition, Health & Aging, 14*(3), 212–217. https://doi.org/10.1007/s12603-010-0052-7

Breijyeh, Z., & Karaman, R. (2020). Comprehensive review on Alzheimer's disease: Causes and treatment. *Molecules, 25*(24), 5789. https://doi.org/10.3390/molecules25245789

Buysse, D. J. (2014). Sleep health: Can we define it? Does it matter? *Sleep, 37*(1), 9–17. https://doi.org/10.5665/sleep.3298

Cappuccio, F. P., D'Elia, L., Strazzullo, P., & Miller, M. A. (2010). Sleep duration and all-cause mortality: A systematic review and meta-analysis of prospective studies. *Sleep, 33*(5), 585–592. https://doi.org/10.1093/sleep/33.5.585

Carnethon, M. R., De Chavez, P. J., Zee, P. C., Kim, K.-Y. A., Liu, K., Goldberger, J. J., Ng, J., & Knutson, K. L. (2016). Disparities in sleep characteristics by race/ethnicity in a population-based sample: Chicago area sleep study. *Sleep Medicine, 18,* 50–55. https://doi.org/10.1016/j.sleep.2015.07.005

Chapman, D. P., Croft, J. B., Liu, Y., Perry, G. S., Presley-Cantrell, L. R., & Ford, E. S. (2013). Excess frequent insufficient sleep in American Indians/Alaska Natives. *Journal of Environmental and Public Health, 2013,* 259645. https://doi.org/10.1155/2013/259645

Chen, J.-H., Waite, L. J., & Lauderdale, D. S. (2015). Marriage, relationship quality, and sleep among U.S. Older adults. *Journal of Health and Social Behavior, 56*(3), 356–377. https://doi.org/10.1177/0022146515594631

Conte, F., Cellini, N., De Rosa, O., Rescott, M. L., Malloggi, S., Giganti, F., & Ficca, G. (2021). The effects of sleep quality on dream and waking emotions. *International Journal of Environmental Research and Public Health, 18*(2), E431. https://doi.org/10.3390/ijerph18020431

Copinschi, G., & Caufriez, A. (2013). Sleep and hormonal changes in aging. *Endocrinology and Metabolism Clinics of North America, 42*(2), 371–389. https://doi.org/10.1016/j.ecl.2013.02.009

Deliens, G., Gilson, M., & Peigneux, P. (2014). Sleep and the processing of emotions. *Experimental Brain Research, 232*(5), 1403–1414. https://doi.org/10.1007/s00221-014-3832-1

Dew, M. A., Hoch, C. C., Buysse, D. J., Monk, T. H., Begley, A. E., Houck, P. R., Hall, M., Kupfer, D. J., & Reynolds, C. F. (2003). Healthy older adults' sleep predicts all-cause mortality at 4 to 19 years of follow-up. *Psychosomatic Medicine, 65*(1), 63–73. https://doi.org/10.1097/01.psy.0000039756.23250.7c

Dong, L., Xie, Y., & Zou, X. (2022). Association between sleep duration and depression in US adults: A cross-sectional study. *Journal of Affective Disorders, 296,* 183–188. https://doi.org/10.1016/j.jad.2021.09.075

Ebben, M. R. (2021). Insomnia: Behavioral treatment in the elderly. *Clinics in Geriatric Medicine, 37*(3), 387–399. https://doi.org/10.1016/j.cger.2021.04.002

Ehlers, C. L., Wills, D. N., Lau, P., & Gilder, D. A. (2017). Sleep quality in an adult American Indian community sample. *Journal of Clinical Sleep Medicine : JCSM : Official Publication of the American Academy of Sleep Medicine, 13*(3), 385–391. https://doi.org/10.5664/jcsm.6486

Elfil, M., Bahbah, E. I., Attia, M. M., Eldokmak, M., & Koo, B. B. (2021). Impact of obstructive sleep Apnea on cognitive and motor functions in Parkinson's disease. *Movement Disorders: Official Journal of the Movement Disorder Society, 36*(3), 570–580. https://doi.org/10.1002/mds.28412

Ellakany, P., Zuñiga, R. A. A., El Tantawi, M., Brown, B., Aly, N. M., Ezechi, O., Uzochukwu, B., Abeldaño, G. F., Ara, E., Ayanore, M. A., Gaffar, B., Al-Khanati, N. M., Ishabiyi, A. O., Jafer, M., Khan, -A. T.-A., Khalid, Z., Lawal, F. B., Lusher, J., Nzimande, N. P., & Folayan, M. O. (2022). Impact of the COVID-19 pandemic on student' sleep patterns, sexual activity, screen use, and food intake: A global survey. *PloS One*, *17*(1), e0262617. https://doi.org/10.1371/journal.pone.0262617

Etholén, A., Pietiläinen, O., Kouvonen, A., Hänninen, M., Rahkonen, O., & Lallukka, T. (2022). Trajectories of insomnia symptoms among aging employees and their associations with memory, learning ability, and concentration after retirement—A prospective Cohort study (2000–2017). *Journal of Aging and Health*, *34* (6–8), 916–928. https://doi.org/10.1177/08982643221078740

Eugene, A. R., & Masiak, J. (2015). The neuroprotective aspects of sleep. *MEDtube Science*, *3*(1), 35–40.

Floyd, J. A., Medler, S. M., Ager, J. W., & Janisse, J. J. (2000). Age-related changes in initiation and maintenance of sleep: A meta-analysis. *Research in Nursing & Health*, *23*(2), 106–117. https://doi.org/10.1002/(sici)1098-240x(200004)23:2<106::aid-nur3>3.0.co;2-a

Foley, D., Ancoli-Israel, S., Britz, P., & Walsh, J. (2004). Sleep disturbances and chronic disease in older adults: Results of the 2003 national sleep foundation sleep in America survey. *Journal of Psychosomatic Research*, *56*(5), 497–502. https://doi.org/10.1016/j.jpsychores.2004.02.010

Foley, D. J., Monjan, A.A., Brown, S. L., Simonsick, E. M., Wallace, R. B., & Blazer, D. G. (1995). Sleep complaints among elderly persons: An epidemiologic study of three communities. *Sleep*, *18*(6), 425–432. https://doi.org/10.1093/sleep/18.6.425

Foley, D. J., Monjan, A. Simonsick, E. M., Wallace, R. B., & Blazer, D. G. (1999). Incidence and remission of insomnia among elderly adults: An epidemiologic study of 6,800 persons over three years. *Sleep*, *22*(Suppl 2), S366–372.

Frank, M. G. (2015). Sleep and synaptic plasticity in the developing and adult brain. *Current Topics in Behavioral Neurosciences*, *25*, 123–149. https://doi.org/10.1007/7854_2014_305

Frank, M. G., & Heller, H. C. (2019). The function(s) of sleep. *Handbook of Experimental Pharmacology*, *253*, 3–34. https://doi.org/10.1007/164_2018_140

Furihata, R., Hall, M. H., Stone, K. L., Ancoli-Israel, S., Smagula, S. F., Cauley, J. A., Kaneita, Y., Uchiyama, M., & Buysse, D. J. Study of Osteoporotic Fractures (SOF) Research Group. (2017). An aggregate measure of sleep health is associated with prevalent and incident clinically significant depression symptoms among community-dwelling older women. *Sleep*, *40*(3). https://doi.org/10.1093/sleep/zsw075.

Gandhi, M. H., & Emmady, P. D. (2022). Physiology, K Complex. *StatPearls*. StatPearls Publishing. http://www.ncbi.nlm.nih.gov/books/NBK557469

Gaspar, L. S., Álvaro, A. R., Moita, J., & Cavadas, C. (2017). Obstructive sleep Apnea and hallmarks of aging. *Trends in Molecular Medicine*, *23*(8), 675–692. https://doi.org/10.1016/j.molmed.2017.06.006

Giuntella, O., Hyde, K., Saccardo, S., & Sadoff, S. (2021). Lifestyle and mental health disruptions during COVID-19. *Proceedings of the National Academy of Sciences*, *118*(9), e2016632118. https://doi.org/10.1073/pnas.2016632118

Gorgoni, M., Lauri, G., Truglia, I., Cordone, S., Sarasso, S., Scarpelli, S., Mangiaruga, A., D'Atri, A., Tempesta, D., Ferrara, M., Marra, C., Rossini, P. M., & De Gennaro, L. (2016). Parietal fast sleep spindle density decrease in Alzheimer's disease and amnesic mild cognitive impairment. *Neural Plasticity*, *2016*, 8376108. https://doi.org/10.1155/2016/8376108

Grandner, M. A. (2017). Sleep, health, and society. *Sleep Medicine Clinics*, *12*(1), 1–22. https://doi.org/10.1016/j.jsmc.2016.10.012

Grandner, M. A., Hale, L., Moore, M., & Patel, N. P. (2010). Mortality associated with short sleep duration: The evidence, the possible mechanisms, and the future. *Sleep Medicine Reviews*, *14*(3), 191–203. https://doi.org/10.1016/j.smrv.2009.07.006

Gulia, K. K., & Kumar, V. M. (2018). Sleep disorders in the elderly: A growing challenge. *Psychogeriatrics: The Official Journal of the Japanese Psychogeriatric Society*, *18*(3), 155–165. https://doi.org/10.1111/psyg.12319

Gupta, R., Grover, S., Basu, A., Krishnan, V., Tripathi, A., Subramanyam, A., Nischal, A., Hussain, A., Mehra, A., Ambekar, A., Saha, G., Mishra, K. K., Bathla, M., Jagiwala, M., Manjunatha, N., Nebhinani, N., Gaur, N., Kumar, N., Dalal, P. K., & Avasthi, A. (2020). Changes in sleep pattern and sleep quality during COVID-19 lockdown. *Indian Journal of Psychiatry*, *62*(4), 370–378. https://doi.org/10.4103/psychiatry.IndianJPsychiatry_523_20

Gureje, O., Kola, L., Ademola, A., & Olley, B. O. (2009). Profile, comorbidity and impact of insomnia in the Ibadan study of ageing. *International Journal of Geriatric Psychiatry*, *24*(7), 686–693. https://doi.org/10.1002/gps.2180

Hepsomali, P., & Groeger, J. A. (2021). Diet, sleep, and mental health: Insights from the UK biobank study. *Nutrients*, *13*(8), 2573. https://doi.org/10.3390/nu13082573

Hot, P., Rauchs, G., Bertran, F., Denise, P., Desgranges, B., Clochon, P., & Eustache, F. (2011). Changes in sleep theta rhythm are related to episodic memory impairment in early Alzheimer's disease. *Biological Psychology*, *87*(3), 334–339. https://doi.org/10.1016/j.biopsycho.2011.04.002

Huang, W.-C., Lin, C.-Y., Togo, F., Lai, T.-F., Liao, Y., Park, J.-H., Hsueh, M.-C., & Park, H. (2021). Association between objectively measured sleep duration and physical function in community-dwelling older adults. *Journal of Clinical Sleep Medicine: JCSM: Official Publication of the American Academy of Sleep Medicine*, *17*(3), 515–520. https://doi.org/10.5664/jcsm.8964

Irwin, M. R. (2015). Why sleep is important for health: A psychoneuroimmunology perspective. *Annual Review of Psychology*, *66*, 143–172. https://doi.org/10.1146/annurev-psych-010213-115205

Jackson, C. L., Powell-Wiley, T. M., Gaston, S. A., Andrews, M. R., Tamura, K., & Ramos, A. (2020). Racial/ Ethnic disparities in sleep health and potential interventions among women in the United States. *Journal of Women's Health (2002)*, *29*(3), 435–442. https://doi.org/10.1089/jwh.2020.8329

Jahrami, H., BaHammam, A. S., Bragazzi, N. L., Saif, Z., Faris, M., & Vitiello, M. V. (2021). Sleep problems during the COVID-19 pandemic by population: A systematic review and meta-analysis. *Journal of Clinical Sleep Medicine: JCSM: Official Publication of the American Academy of Sleep Medicine*, *17*(2), 299–313. https://doi.org/10.5664/jcsm.8930

Johnson, D. A., Jackson, C. L., Williams, N. J., & Alcántara, C. (2019). Are sleep patterns influenced by race/ ethnicity - a marker of relative advantage or disadvantage? Evidence to date. *Nature and Science of Sleep*, *11*, 79–95. https://doi.org/10.2147/NSS.S169312

Knutson, K. L. (2010). Sleep duration and cardiometabolic risk: A review of the epidemiologic evidence. *Best Practice & Research. Clinical Endocrinology & Metabolism*, *24*(5), 731–743. https://doi.org/10.1016/j. beem.2010.07.001

Kocevska, D., Lysen, T. S., Dotinga, A., Koopman-Verhoeff, M. E., Luijk, M. P. C. M., Antypa, N., Biermasz, N. R., Blokstra, A., Brug, J., Burk, W. J., Comijs, H. C., Corpeleijn, E., Dashti, H. S., de Bruin, E. J., de Graaf, R., Derks, I. P. M., Dewald-Kaufmann, J. F., Elders, P. J. M., Gemke, R. J. B. J., & Tiemeier, H. (2021). Sleep characteristics across the lifespan in 1.1 million people from the Netherlands, United Kingdom and United States: A systematic review and meta-analysis. *Nature Human Behaviour*, *5*(1). Article 1. https://doi. org/10.1038/s41562-020-00965-x

Kripke, D. F., Garfinkel, L., Wingard, D. L., Klauber, M. R., & Marler, M. R. (2002). Mortality associated with sleep duration and insomnia. *Archives of General Psychiatry*, *59*(2), 131–136. https://doi.org/10.1001/ archpsyc.59.2.131

Kryger, M. H., Roth, T., & Dement, W. C. (2017). Principles and practice of sleep medicine. Elsevier. /z-wcorg/. https://TB4CZ3EN3E.search.serialssolutions.com/?sid=sersol&SS_jc=TC0001631362&title=Principles%20 and%20practice%20of%20sleep%20medicine

Laugsand, L. E., Vatten, L. J., Platou, C., & Janszky, I. (2011). Insomnia and the risk of acute myocardial infarction: A population study. *Circulation*, *124*(19), 2073–2081. https://doi.org/10.1161/CIRCULATIONAHA. 111.025858

LeBlanc, M., Mérette, C., Savard, J., Ivers, H., Baillargeon, L., & Morin, C. M. (2009). Incidence and risk factors of insomnia in a population-based sample. *Sleep*, *32*(8), 1027–1037. https://doi.org/10.1093/sleep/32.8.1027

Lewis, L. D. (2021). The interconnected causes and consequences of sleep in the brain. *Science (New York, N.Y.)*, *374*(6567), 564–568. https://doi.org/10.1126/science.abi8375

Li, J., Vitiello, M. V., & Gooneratne, N. (2018). Sleep in normal aging. *Sleep Medicine Clinics*, *13*(1), 1–11. https://doi.org/10.1016/j.jsmc.2017.09.001

Liguori, C., Mercuri, N. B., Nuccetelli, M., Izzi, F., Cordella, A., Bernardini, S., & Placidi, F. (2019). Obstructive sleep apnea may induce orexinergic system and cerebral β-amyloid metabolism dysregulation: Is it a further proof for Alzheimer's disease risk? *Sleep Medicine*, *56*, 171–176. https://doi.org/10.1016/j.sleep.2019.01.003

Liguori, C., Placidi, F., Izzi, F., Spanetta, M., Mercuri, N. B., & Di Pucchio, A. (2020). Sleep dysregulation, memory impairment, and CSF biomarkers during different levels of neurocognitive functioning in Alzheimer's disease course. *Alzheimer's Research & Therapy*, *12*(1), 5. https://doi.org/10.1186/s13195-019-0571-3

Liu, S., Pan, J., Tang, K., Lei, Q., He, L., Meng, Y., Cai, X., & Li, Z. (2020). Sleep spindles, K-complexes, limb movements and sleep stage proportions may be biomarkers for amnestic mild cognitive impairment and Alzheimer's disease. *Sleep & Breathing = Schlaf & Atmung*, *24*(2), 637–651. https://doi.org/10.1007/ s11325-019-01970-9

Liu, Y., Wheaton, A. G., Chapman, D. P., Cunningham, T. J., Lu, H., & Croft, J. B. (2016). Prevalence of healthy sleep duration among adults—United States, 2014. *MMWR. Morbidity and Mortality Weekly Report, 65*(6), 137–141. https://doi.org/10.15585/mmwr.mm6506a1

Lo, J. C., Groeger, J. A., Cheng, G. H., Dijk, D.-J., & Chee, M. W. L. (2016). Self-reported sleep duration and cognitive performance in older adults: A systematic review and meta-analysis. *Sleep Medicine, 17*, 87–98. https://doi.org/10.1016/j.sleep.2015.08.021

Lovato, N., Lack, L., Wright, H., & Kennaway, D. J. (2014). Evaluation of a brief treatment program of cognitive behavior therapy for insomnia in older adults. *Sleep, 37*(1), 117–126. https://doi.org/10.5665/sleep.3320

Luo, J., Zhu, G., Zhao, Q., Guo, Q., Meng, H., Hong, Z., & Ding, D. (2013). Prevalence and risk factors of poor sleep quality among Chinese elderly in an urban community: Results from the Shanghai aging study. *PloS One, 8*(11), e81261. https://doi.org/10.1371/journal.pone.0081261

Lysen, T. S., Darweesh, S. K. L., Ikram, M. K., Luik, A. I., & Ikram, M. A. (2019). Sleep and risk of parkinsonism and Parkinson's disease: A population-based study. *Brain: A Journal of Neurology, 142*(7), 2013–2022. https://doi.org/10.1093/brain/awz113

Maggi, G., Trojano, L., Barone, P., & Santangelo, G. (2021). Sleep disorders and cognitive dysfunctions in Parkinson's disease: A meta-analytic study. *Neuropsychology Review, 31*(4), 643–682. https://doi.org/10.1007/s11065-020-09473-1

Mallon, L., Broman, J. E., & Hetta, J. (2002). Sleep complaints predict coronary artery disease mortality in males: A 12-year follow-up study of a middle-aged Swedish population. *Journal of Internal Medicine, 251*(3), 207–216. https://doi.org/10.1046/j.1365-2796.2002.00941.x

Mamalaki, E., Tsapanou, A., Anastasiou, C. A., Kosmidis, M. H., Dardiotis, E., Hadjigeorgiou, G. M., Sakka, P., Scarmeas, N., & Yannakoulia, M. (2019). Associations between sleep and obesity indices in older adults: Results from the HELIAD study. *Aging Clinical and Experimental Research, 31*(11), 1645–1650. https://doi.org/10.1007/s40520-018-01113-2

Markun, L. C., & Sampat, A. (2020). Clinician-focused overview and developments in polysomnography. *Current Sleep Medicine Reports, 6*(4), 309–321. https://doi.org/10.1007/s40675-020-00197-5

Matricciani, L., Olds, T., & Petkov, J. (2012). In search of lost sleep: Secular trends in the sleep time of school-aged children and adolescents. *Sleep Medicine Reviews, 16*(3), 203–211. https://doi.org/10.1016/j.smrv.2011.03.005

Mattis, J., & Sehgal, A. (2016). Circadian rhythms, sleep, and disorders of aging. *Trends in Endocrinology and Metabolism: TEM, 27*(4), 192–203. https://doi.org/10.1016/j.tem.2016.02.003

Milligan, S. A., & Chesson, A. L. (2002). Restless legs syndrome in the older adult: Diagnosis and management. *Drugs & Aging, 19*(10), 741–751. https://doi.org/10.2165/00002512-200219100-00003

Milojevich, H. M., & Lukowski, A. F. (2016). Sleep and mental health in undergraduate students with generally healthy sleep habits. *PloS One, 11*(6), e0156372. https://doi.org/10.1371/journal.pone.0156372

Miner, B., & Kryger, M. H. (2017). Sleep in the aging population. *Sleep Medicine Clinics, 12*(1), 31–38. https://doi.org/10.1016/j.jsmc.2016.10.008

Morgan, K., Gregory, P., Tomeny, M., David, B. M., & Gascoigne, C. (2012). Self-help treatment for insomnia symptoms associated with chronic conditions in older adults: A randomized controlled trial. *Journal of the American Geriatrics Society, 60*(10), 1803–1810. https://doi.org/10.1111/j.1532-5415.2012.04175.x

Morgenthaler, T. I., Owens, J., Alessi, C., Boehlecke, B., Brown, T. M., Coleman, J., Friedman, L., Kapur, V. K., Lee-Chiong, T., Pancer, J., & Swick, T. J. American Academy of Sleep Medicine. (2006). Practice parameters for behavioral treatment of bedtime problems and night wakings in infants and young children. *Sleep, 29*(10), 1277–1281.

Morin, C. M., Colecchi, C., Stone, J., Sood, R., & Brink, D. (1999). Behavioral and pharmacological therapies for late-life insomnia: A randomized controlled trial. *JAMA, 281*(11), 991–999. https://doi.org/10.1001/jama.281.11.991

Mullins, A. E., Kam, K., Parekh, A., Bubu, O. M., Osorio, R. S., & Varga, A. W. (2020). Obstructive sleep apnea and its treatment in aging: Effects on Alzheimer's disease biomarkers, cognition, brain structure and neurophysiology. *Neurobiology of Disease, 145*, 105054. https://doi.org/10.1016/j.nbd.2020.105054

Murillo-Rodriguez, E., Arias-Carrion, O., Zavala-Garcia, A., Sarro-Ramirez, A., Huitron-Resendiz, S., & Arankowsky-Sandoval, G. (2012). Basic sleep mechanisms: An integrative review. *Central Nervous System Agents in Medicinal Chemistry, 12*(1), 38–54. https://doi.org/10.2174/187152412800229107

Nakazaki, C., Noda, A., Koike, Y., Yamada, S., Murohara, T., & Ozaki, N. (2012). Association of insomnia and short sleep duration with atherosclerosis risk in the elderly. *American Journal of Hypertension*, *25*(11), 1149–1155. https://doi.org/10.1038/ajh.2012.107

Ohayon, M. M., Carskadon, M. A., Guilleminault, C., & Vitiello, M. V. (2004). Meta-analysis of quantitative sleep parameters from childhood to old age in healthy individuals: Developing normative sleep values across the human lifespan. *Sleep*, *27*(7), 1255–1273. https://doi.org/10.1093/sleep/27.7.1255

Ohayon, M. M., & Vecchierini, M.-F. (2005). Normative sleep data, cognitive function and daily living activities in older adults in the community. *Sleep*, *28*(8), 981–989.

Okoye, S. M., Szanton, S. L., Perrin, N. A., Nkimbeng, M., Schrack, J. A., Han, H.-R., Nyhuis, C., Wanigatunga, S., & Spira, A. P. (2021). Objectively measured sleep and physical function: Associations in low-income older adults with disabilities. *Sleep Health*, *7*(6), 735–741. https://doi.org/10.1016/j.sleh.2021.09.001

Okuro, M., & Morimoto, S. (2014). Sleep apnea in the elderly. *Current Opinion in Psychiatry*, *27*(6), 472–477. https://doi.org/10.1097/YCO.0000000000000105

Omvik, S., Sivertsen, B., Pallesen, S., Bjorvatn, B., Havik, O. E., & Nordhus, I. H. (2008). Daytime functioning in older patients suffering from chronic insomnia: Treatment outcome in a randomized controlled trial comparing CBT with Zopiclone. *Behaviour Research and Therapy*, *46*(5), 623–641. https://doi.org/10.1016/j.brat.2008.02.013

Pace-Schott, E. F., & Spencer, R. M. C. (2015). Sleep-dependent memory consolidation in healthy aging and mild cognitive impairment. *Current Topics in Behavioral Neurosciences*, *25*, 307–330. https://doi.org/10.1007/7854_2014_300

Palmer, C. A., & Alfano, C. A. (2017). Sleep and emotion regulation: An organizing, integrative review. *Sleep Medicine Reviews*, *31*, 6–16. https://doi.org/10.1016/j.smrv.2015.12.006

Parthasarathy, S., Vasquez, M. M., Halonen, M., Bootzin, R., Quan, S. F., Martinez, F. D., & Guerra, S. (2015). Persistent Insomnia is associated with mortality risk. *The American Journal of Medicine*, *128*(3), 268–275.e2. https://doi.org/10.1016/j.amjmed.2014.10.015

Peppard, P. E., Young, T., Barnet, J. H., Palta, M., Hagen, E. W., & Hla, K. M. (2013). Increased prevalence of sleep-disordered breathing in adults. *American Journal of Epidemiology*, *177*(9), 1006–1014. https://doi.org/10.1093/aje/kws342

Poewe, W., Seppi, K., Tanner, C. M., Halliday, G. M., Brundin, P., Volkmann, J., Schrag, A.-E., & Lang, A. E. (2017). Parkinson disease. *Nature Reviews Disease Primers*, *3*(1). Article 1. https://doi.org/10.1038/nrdp.2017.13

Pótári, A., Ujma, P. P., Konrad, B. N., Genzel, L., Simor, P., Körmendi, J., Gombos, F., Steiger, A., Dresler, M., & Bódizs, R. (2017). Age-related changes in sleep EEG are attenuated in highly intelligent individuals. *NeuroImage*, *146*, 554–560. https://doi.org/10.1016/j.neuroimage.2016.09.039

Ramos Socarras, L., Potvin, J., & Forest, G. (2021). COVID-19 and sleep patterns in adolescents and young adults. *Sleep Medicine*, *83*, 26–33. https://doi.org/10.1016/j.sleep.2021.04.010

Reda, F., Gorgoni, M., Lauri, G., Truglia, I., Cordone, S., Scarpelli, S., Mangiaruga, A., D'Atri, A., Ferrara, M., Lacidogna, G., Marra, C., Rossini, P. M., & De Gennaro, L. (2017). In search of sleep biomarkers of Alzheimer's disease: K-complexes do not discriminate between patients with mild cognitive impairment and healthy controls. *Brain Sciences*, *7*(5), E51. https://doi.org/10.3390/brainsci7050051

Robbins, R., DiClemente, R. J. J., Troxel, A., Rapoport, D., Rogers, A., Donley, T., Osorio, R., & Jean-Louis, G. (2019). 0693 Examining disparities in sleep health (duration and Quality) Among black and white older adults in the U.S.: An analysis from the national health and aging trends study (nhats). *Sleep*, *42*(Suppl._1), A278. https://doi.org/10.1093/sleep/zsz067.691

Robbins, R., Quan, S. F., Buysse, D. J., Weaver, M. D., Walker, M. P., Drake, C. L., Monten, K., Barger, L. K., Rajaratnam, S. M. W., Roth, T., & Czeisler, C. A. (2022). A nationally representative survey assessing restorative sleep in US adults. *Frontiers in Sleep*, *1*. https://www.frontiersin.org/articles/10.3389/frsle.2022.935228

Robbins, R., Quan, S. F., Weaver, M. D., Bormes, G., Barger, L. K., & Czeisler, C. A. (2021). Examining sleep deficiency and disturbance and their risk for incident dementia and all-cause mortality in older adults across 5 years in the United States. *Aging*, *13*(3), 3254–3268. https://doi.org/10.18632/aging.202591

Robbins, R., Trinh-Shevrin, C., Chong, S. K., Chanko, N., Diaby, F., Quan, S. F., & Kwon, S. C. (2022). Examining demographic, work, and sleep characteristics among older South Asian American yellow taxi drivers in New York City: A brief report. *Sleep Medicine*, *96*, 128–131. https://doi.org/10.1016/j.sleep.2022.04.012

Rosenberg, R. S., & Van Hout, S. (2014). The American academy of sleep medicine inter-scorer reliability program: Respiratory events. *Journal of Clinical Sleep Medicine*, *10*(4), 447–454. https://doi.org/10.5664/jcsm.3630

Rybarczyk, B., Stepanski, E., Fogg, L., Lopez, M., Barry, P., & Davis, A. (2005). A placebo-controlled test of cognitive-behavioral therapy for comorbid insomnia in older adults. *Journal of Consulting and Clinical Psychology, 73*(6), 1164–1174. https://doi.org/10.1037/0022-006X.73.6.1164

Sadler, P., McLaren, S., Klein, B., Harvey, J., & Jenkins, M. (2018). Cognitive behavior therapy for older adults with insomnia and depression: A randomized controlled trial in community mental health services. *Sleep, 41*(8). https://doi.org/10.1093/sleep/zsy104

Sateia, M. J., Buysse, D. J., Krystal, A. D., Neubauer, D. N., & Heald, J. L. (2017). Clinical practice guideline for the pharmacologic treatment of chronic insomnia in adults: An American academy of sleep medicine clinical practice guideline. *Journal of Clinical Sleep Medicine: JCSM: Official Publication of the American Academy of Sleep Medicine, 13*(2), 307–349. https://doi.org/10.5664/jcsm.6470

Schneider, L. (2020). Neurobiology and neuroprotective benefits of sleep. *Continuum (Minneapolis, Minn.), 26*(4), 848–870. https://doi.org/10.1212/CON.0000000000000878

Schroeck, J. L., Ford, J., Conway, E. L., Kurtzhalts, K. E., Gee, M. E., Vollmer, K. A., & Mergenhagen, K. A. (2016). Review of safety and efficacy of sleep medicines in older adults. *Clinical Therapeutics, 38*(11), 2340–2372. https://doi.org/10.1016/j.clinthera.2016.09.010

Scott, A. J., Webb, T. L., Martyn-St James, M., Rowse, G., & Weich, S. (2021). Improving sleep quality leads to better mental health: A meta-analysis of randomised controlled trials. *Sleep Medicine Reviews, 60*, 101556. https://doi.org/10.1016/j.smrv.2021.101556

Scullin, M. K., & Bliwise, D. L. (2015). Sleep, cognition, and normal aging: Integrating a half century of multidisciplinary research. *Perspectives on Psychological Science: A Journal of the Association for Psychological Science, 10*(1), 97–137. https://doi.org/10.1177/1745691614556680

Sheehan, C., & Iida, M. (2021). Spousal educational attainment and sleep duration among American older adults. *The Journals of Gerontology. Series B, Psychological Sciences and Social Sciences, 76*(5), 1015–1026. https://doi.org/10.1093/geronb/gbaa206

Shen, L., van Schie, J., Ditchburn, G., Brook, L., & Bei, B. (2018). Positive and negative emotions: Differential associations with sleep duration and quality in adolescents. *Journal of Youth and Adolescence, 47*(12), 2584–2595. https://doi.org/10.1007/s10964-018-0899-1

Shi, L., Chen, S.-J., Ma, M.-Y., Bao, Y.-P., Han, Y., Wang, Y.-M., Shi, J., Vitiello, M. V., & Lu, L. (2018). Sleep disturbances increase the risk of dementia: A systematic review and meta-analysis. *Sleep Medicine Reviews, 40*, 4–16. https://doi.org/10.1016/j.smrv.2017.06.010

Siciliano, M., Trojano, L., Santangelo, G., De Micco, R., Tedeschi, G., & Tessitore, A. (2018). Fatigue in Parkinson's disease: A systematic review and meta-analysis. *Movement Disorders: Official Journal of the Movement Disorder Society, 33*(11), 1712–1723. https://doi.org/10.1002/mds.27461

Sivertsen, B., Omvik, S., Pallesen, S., Bjorvatn, B., Havik, O. E., Kvale, G., Nielsen, G. H., & Nordhus, I. H. (2006). Cognitive behavioral therapy vs zopiclone for treatment of chronic primary insomnia in older adults: A randomized controlled trial. *JAMA, 295*(24), 2851–2858. https://doi.org/10.1001/jama.295.24.2851

Stone, K. L., Ensrud, K. E., & Ancoli-Israel, S. (2008). Sleep, insomnia and falls in elderly patients. *Sleep Medicine, 9*(Suppl 1), S18–22. https://doi.org/10.1016/S1389-9457(08)70012-1

Tai, X. Y., Chen, C., Manohar, S., & Husain, M. (2022). Impact of sleep duration on executive function and brain structure. *Communications Biology, 5*(1). Article 1. https://doi.org/10.1038/s42003-022-03123-3

Tempesta, D., Socci, V., De Gennaro, L., & Ferrara, M. (2018). Sleep and emotional processing. *Sleep Medicine Reviews, 40*, 183–195. https://doi.org/10.1016/j.smrv.2017.12.005

Trotti, L. M., & Becker, L. A. (2019). Iron for the treatment of restless legs syndrome. *Cochrane Database of Systematic Reviews, 1*. https://doi.org/10.1002/14651858.CD007834.pub3

Van Cauter, E., Leproult, R., & Plat, L. (2000). Age-related changes in slow wave sleep and REM sleep and relationship with growth hormone and cortisol levels in healthy men. *JAMA, 284*(7), 861–868. https://doi.org/10.1001/jama.284.7.861

van Coevorden, A., Mockel, J., Laurent, E., Kerkhofs, M., L'Hermite-Balériaux, M., Decoster, C., Nève, P., & Van Cauter, E. (1991). Neuroendocrine rhythms and sleep in aging men. *The American Journal of Physiology, 260*(4 Pt 1), E651–661. https://doi.org/10.1152/ajpendo.1991.260.4.E651

Vanderlinden, J., Boen, F., & van Uffelen, J. G. Z. (2020). Effects of physical activity programs on sleep outcomes in older adults: A systematic review. *The International Journal of Behavioral Nutrition and Physical Activity, 17*(1), 11. https://doi.org/10.1186/s12966-020-0913-3

Vaughan, C. P., & Bliwise, D. L. (2018). Sleep and Nocturia in older adults. *Sleep Medicine Clinics, 13*(1), 107–116. https://doi.org/10.1016/j.jsmc.2017.09.010

Vgontzas, A. N., Fernandez-Mendoza, J., Liao, D., & Bixler, E. O. (2013). Insomnia with objective short sleep duration: The most biologically severe phenotype of the disorder. *Sleep Medicine Reviews*, *17*(4), 241–254. https://doi.org/10.1016/j.smrv.2012.09.005

Vitiello, M. V., Larsen, L. H., & Moe, K. E. (2004). Age-related sleep change: Gender and estrogen effects on the subjective-objective sleep quality relationships of healthy, noncomplaining older men and women. *Journal of Psychosomatic Research*, *56*(5), 503–510. https://doi.org/10.1016/S0022-3999(04)00023-6

Walker, M. P. (2009). The role of sleep in cognition and emotion. *Annals of the New York Academy of Sciences*, *1156*, 168–197. https://doi.org/10.1111/j.1749-6632.2009.04416.x

Wei, J., Hou, R., Xie, L., Chandrasekar, E. K., Lu, H., Wang, T., Li, C., & Xu, H. (2021). Sleep, sedentary activity, physical activity, and cognitive function among older adults: The National Health and Nutrition Examination Survey, 2011–2014. *Journal of Science and Medicine in Sport*, *24*(2), 189–194. https://doi.org/10.1016/j.jsams.2020.09.013

Whinnery, J., Jackson, N., Rattanaumpawan, P., & Grandner, M. A. (2014). Short and long sleep duration associated with race/ethnicity, sociodemographics, and socioeconomic position. *Sleep*, *37*(3), 601–611. https://doi.org/10.5665/sleep.3508

Widiger, T. A., Costa, P. T., & Association, A. P. (2013). Personality disorders and the five-factor model of personality. JSTOR.

Worley, S. L. (2018). The extraordinary importance of sleep. *Pharmacy and Therapeutics*, *43*(12), 758–763.

Xie, L., Kang, H., Xu, Q., Chen, M. J., Liao, Y., Thiyagarajan, M., O'Donnell, J., Christensen, D. J., Nicholson, C., Iliff, J. J., Takano, T., Deane, R., & Nedergaard, M. (2013). Sleep drives metabolite clearance from the adult brain. *Science (New York, N.Y.)*, *342*(6156). https://doi.org/10.1126/science.1241224

Yin, Y., Liu, Y., Pan, X., Chen, R., Li, P., Wu, H.-J., Zhao, Z.-Q., Li, Y.-P., Huang, L.-Q., Zhuang, J.-H., & Zhao, Z.-X. (2016). Interleukin-1β Promoter polymorphism enhances the risk of sleep disturbance in Alzheimer's disease. *PloS One*, *11*(3), e0149945. https://doi.org/10.1371/journal.pone.0149945

Yip, T., & Cheon, Y. M. (2020). Sleep, psychopathology and cultural diversity. *Current Opinion in Psychology*, *34*, 123–127. https://doi.org/10.1016/j.copsyc.2020.02.006

Yuan, R. K., Zitting, K.-M., Maskati, L., & Huang, J. (2022). Increased sleep duration and delayed sleep timing during the COVID-19 pandemic. *Scientific Reports*, *12*(1), 10937. https://doi.org/10.1038/s41598-022-14782-x

Zhang, Y., Ren, R., Sanford, L. D., Yang, L., Zhou, J., Tan, L., Li, T., Zhang, J., Wing, Y.-K., Shi, J., Lu, L., & Tang, X. (2020). Sleep in Parkinson's disease: A systematic review and meta-analysis of polysomnographic findings. *Sleep Medicine Reviews*, *51*, 101281. https://doi.org/10.1016/j.smrv.2020.101281

Zhang, Y., Ren, R., Yang, L., Zhang, H., Shi, Y., Okhravi, H. R., Vitiello, M. V., Sanford, L. D., & Tang, X. (2022). Sleep in Alzheimer's disease: A systematic review and meta-analysis of polysomnographic findings. *Translational Psychiatry*, *12*(1), 136. https://doi.org/10.1038/s41398-022-01897-y

CHAPTER

EMERGING RESEARCH IN AGING AND ALZHEIMER'S DISEASE AND ALZHEIMER'S DISEASE-RELATED DEMENTIAS

KOMAL PATEL MURALI, KALISHA BONDS JOHNSON, ABRAHAM AIZER BRODY

LEARNING OBJECTIVES

By the end of this chapter, readers will be able to:

- Elucidate emerging challenges in care partner and caregiver research that are influenced by health inequities and systematic racism and bias.

- Understand current challenges in effectively implementing technology solutions in an equitable fashion to address care for persons living with dementia and their care partners.

- Consider how multimorbidity and serious illness should be integrated into research involving persons living with dementia and their care partners.

INTRODUCTION

Within the context of aging and the disease trajectory of Alzheimer's disease and Alzheimer's disease-related dementias (AD/ADRD), there are both opportunities and challenges in emerging research. Four emerging areas that require specific focus and understanding include: 1) caregiving and dyadic research; 2) multimorbidity and serious illness; 3) palliative care; and 4) the use of technology. While each of these four areas merits further study with respect to the entire population of dementia-impacted individuals in the United States, special focus must be accorded to diverse and historically underserved populations of persons living with dementia, as extant research has largely ignored the unique attributes and needs of racial and ethnic minoritized groups and low-income populations.

AD/ADRD is characterized by progressive worsening cognitive and behavioral symptoms that require substantial reliance on a care partner or family member for both activities of daily living (ADL, basic self-care tasks that all individuals must complete to maintain health) and instrumental activities of daily living (IADL, tasks that require complex thinking and are essential to one's ability to live independently, such as organizational skills) (Shin & Habermann, 2022). For this reason, AD/ADRD research, unlike other aging research, has focused heavily on understanding the caregiving experiences of care partners of persons living with dementia. Indeed, early AD/ADRD research often neglected to include the perspectives of people living with AD/ADRD for fear that they may be unable to accurately answer questions or fully participate in research. However, recent evidence has supported the inclusion of persons living with dementia, especially those in the mild to moderate stages of illness (Bonds et al., 2020; Lyons et al., 2002).

This chapter discusses both challenges and emerging opportunities in AD/ADRD research focused on caregiving dyads, multimorbidity and serious illness, and technology.

CAREGIVING AND DYADIC RESEARCH

Persons living with dementia and their care partners often make decisions together as a dyad, which is a key area for improving care in this population. The surge of dyadic research in AD/ADRD has brought new opportunities as well as challenges. For example, hearing the voices of both members of the dyad allows researchers to examine personal and interpersonal factors impacting disease expression (Bonds Johnson, Epps et al., 2021), including a diverse range of experiences that encompass both living with the disease as well as caregiving for people living with the disease. Dyadic research evidence offers robust data for the development and design of interventions that can be beneficial for improving outcomes and delivery of high-quality care that responds to the needs of both members of the dyad (Whitlatch et al., 2006).

However, designing and implementing dyadic caregiving research is challenging. First, dual eligibility is required in research, which means both the person living with AD/ADRD and their care partner must screen for eligibility to participate (Szabo et al., 2016). Careful consideration of inclusion and exclusion criteria is warranted to maximize the opportunities to recruit. Second, measures and recruitment materials must consider the member of the dyad with whom it is engaging because dyadic multilevel modeling (e.g., Actor-Partner Interdependence Modeling) (Cook & Kenny, 2005; Lyons & Lee,

2020) often requires the use of parallel scales. Parallel scales are separate instruments for the person living with AD/ADRD as well as the care partner. For example, the Dyadic Relationship Scale (Sebern & Whitlatch, 2007), is a good example of a parallel scale; it has a scale for the person living with AD/ADRD as well as the care partner. Not all scales will work as parallel scales, which should be thought out before determining the measures used in a dyadic study. For qualitative research, one must decide whether interviews will occur together or separately, and a strong rationale is needed for why. If the research is focused on recruiting underrepresented racial and ethnic dyads, there may also be a need to linguistically and culturally tailor the study design to the population of interest (Parker et al., 2022).

As older adults live longer, the racial and ethnic makeup of the United States (US) population is evolving. With this evolution, differences are emerging in who is providing care for these older adults. African American (Black) older adults have more than double the prevalence of AD/ADRD compared to non-Hispanic White (White) older adults and Hispanic (Latine) older adults have one and half times the prevalence of AD/ADRD compared to White older adults (Alzheimer's Association, 2022). These prevalence figures offer an indication of the disproportionate burden of AD/ADRD caregiving among Black and Latine Americans. Yet, these and other minoritized populations, including Asian American, Native Hawaiian and Pacific Islander (NH/PI), and American Indian/Alaskan Native (AI/AN) people, are often underrepresented in AD/ADRD research, generally, and in caregiving and dyadic research, specifically. Developing culturally and linguistically tailored recruitment and retention methods could support increased participation by individuals from these groups that could better inform interventions for caregivers of diverse backgrounds (Hu et al., 2021; Ta Park et al., 2021).

Recently, researchers have begun examining outcomes related to aging and AD/ADRD within Black and White communities, highlighting the importance of life course factors, social determinants of health (SDOH), and cultural nuances. That is, only in recent years have researchers begun developing studies that are centered on the lived experiences of these racial and ethnic groups without comparing their experiences to White older adults (Bonds Johnson, Brewster et al., 2021).

Measuring life course factors has created new challenges and opportunities in research. For example, in earlier studies, heterogeneity in Black older adults' educational status was described by their completed grade level. Research has recently highlighted capturing educational status by collecting data on educational quality, which captures the amount of time spent in the classroom with less focus on the grade level achieved (Sisco et al., 2015). As a result, the differences identified in cognitive decline of Black older adults was better explained by educational quality than completed grade level, highlighting the need to look beyond completed grade level when conducting research.

Shared decision-making is another area in which research is evolving. Previously, shared decision-making focused on the process that occurs between a patient and their health care provider that produces a mutually agreed-upon pathway regarding care and treatment. Shared decision-making has been shown to be effective in building rapport between patients and providers, contributing to improved patient satisfaction (Makoul & Clayman, 2006; Shay & Lafata, 2015). Within the context of dementia, however, shared decision-making must focus not only on the process that occurs between provider and patient, but also on understanding the care preferences of the dyad involved in the dementia experience – i.e., the person living with AD/ADRD and their principal care partner or caregiver. Emerging research in AD/ADRD is expanding the concept of shared decision-making to this triad of patient, provider, and care partner (Bonds Johnson, Epps et al., 2021).

MULTIMORBIDITY AND SERIOUS ILLNESS

Multimorbidity

Persons living with dementia often have comorbid illness or multimorbidity (Snowden et al., 2017). Typically, multimorbidity is defined as an individual having two or more chronic conditions for which they require regular medical care and result in ADL limitations (Grembowski et al., 2014; Murali et al., 2020). For persons living with dementia, multimorbidity occurs when concurrent diagnoses such as congestive heart failure, cancer, or lung disease are also present. Having multimorbid conditions can result in an individual living with dementia developing an increased risk of disability, mortality, and caregiver strain (Mitchell, 2015).

More specifically, multimorbidity among persons living with dementia has been shown to increase the likelihood of unwanted hospitalizations, traumatic and costly transitions between health care settings, and untimely institutionalization in nursing homes or long-term care facilities (Amjad et al., 2019; Mitchell et al., 2009). The cumulative effect of multiple chronic conditions on individuals living with AD/ADRD necessitates tailored multidisciplinary care to meet the complex needs of these individuals across health care settings, including hospitals and health centers as well as in-home care and community-based settings (Murali et al., 2021; Ploeg et al., 2020; Sadarangani et al., 2022). These needs include managing symptoms, compensating for functional impairment, coordinating care, facilitating care conversations, and managing medications to mitigate adverse outcomes. Ensuring that patients and care partners have support from a skilled care team that understands patients' medical needs and life experiences and prioritizes patient- and family-centered care is critical to avoiding care partner strain and providing quality care across health care settings (Gilmore-Bykovskyi et al., 2017).

Toward this end, future research should prioritize the development of innovative care models that effectively meet the needs of persons living with dementia and multimorbidity across health care settings. Including multiple stakeholders in AD/ADRD research, such as health care organizations, patients, care partners, and clinicians, will be critical to developing a comprehensive understanding of the existing health care system – including both its challenges and strengths – so that innovative, responsive, effective care delivery models can be integrated within it. Novel approaches for provision of AD/ADRD care that are culturally and linguistically tailored to the needs of racially and ethnically diverse persons living with dementia are also needed. However, in order to develop evidence-based approaches for these populations, increasing the recruitment and retention of racially and ethnically diverse persons living with dementia and multimorbidity in clinical trials is needed to identify existing gaps and develop tailored culturally sensitive approaches for dementia care across all stages of illness (Gilmore-Bykovskyi et al., 2019).

Serious Illness

Distinct from multimorbidity, serious illness refers to a later phase of the disease experience wherein individuals develop greater risk for high symptom burden, poor or compro-
mised quality of life, functional impairment, and increased health care utilization and costs – all
of which contribute to greater caregiver burden and stress (Kelley, 2014). As persons living
with dementia progress along the serious illness trajectory, specifically for those with moderate to severe AD/ADRD, worsening physical and cognitive function create a high-acuity
care situation in the home prior to end-of-life care, a responsibility that often falls on family
and friends who serve as caregivers or care partners (Aldridge et al., 2022; Amjad et al.,
2019; Mitchell, 2015). In fact, many persons living with dementia and multimorbidity frequently face frail or fragile health status, requiring daily caregiving assistance in the home
and worsening physical or cognitive decline that can require a transition to a nursing home
or assisted living. The cumulative impact of serious illness, multimorbidity, and AD/ADRD
can significantly affect quality of care and result in poor outcomes; therefore, optimizing
care strategies to improve care for this population is an emerging area of research in need
of innovative solutions.

Establishing a better understanding of health care utilization and transitions among
people living with dementia is critical to improving care strategies. In moderate to severe
AD/ADRD, research has shown that individuals may experience a greater likelihood of
increased use of acute care services, poor end-of-life care outcomes, and burdensome or
aggressive care that may be misaligned with patient and family values and preferences
(Gilmore-Bykovskyi et al., 2017; Harrison et al., 2022; Lin et al., 2022). Yet, the events that
lead to these significant points along the serious illness trajectory have not yet been well
described in the literature, particularly for racially and ethnically minoritized populations.
A better understanding of these transition points could help researchers to develop and test
preventive and supportive strategies prior to patients requiring acute help in institutional
settings. In the context of worsening behavioral or psychological symptoms, which may be
compounded by the difficult physical manifestations of multimorbidity, hospitalizations are
more likely to occur if a care partner or family member experiences distress and is unable
to safely manage symptoms at home (Maust et al., 2017). Often, unintended and potentially
avoidable hospitalizations and adverse events are more likely to occur in this population as
a result (Maust et al., 2019).

Developing a robust dementia care workforce is another key area of interest. Providing
high-quality AD/ADRD care for persons with dementia and multimorbidity – particularly
as they progress along the trajectory of serious illness – is essential to ensuring quality of
life for these patients and requires the training, preparation, and collaborative work of paid
and unpaid caregivers as well as health care professionals. As the prevalence of dementia in
the older adult population increases and as the population of people living with dementia
diversifies, existing care delivery models and health care systems will require integration of
dementia-focused care delivered by a well-prepared interdisciplinary, multicultural, and
multilinguistic workforce (National Academy of Sciences, 2021). The training of care partners, family members, and interdisciplinary health care workers should be prioritized for
ensuring optimal patient and family-centered care delivery for persons living with dementia
to manage the complex care needs of persons living with dementia and multimorbidity
(Burgdorf et al., 2021; Murali et al., 2022). Recruiting, training, and retaining people in the

professional and paraprofessional workforce from the racial and ethnic minoritized communities that are disproportionately impacted by dementia prevalence, and in which incidence is increasing most rapidly, must be a priority. Furthermore, future research must focus on examining optimal care delivery mechanisms for seriously ill persons living with dementia across health care settings. Given the limited extant evidence in this area, engaging the affected population and their care partners in clinical research remains an ongoing imperative for dementia care science. Furthermore, more randomized clinical trials and embedded pragmatic trials, particularly in the community, are needed to identify effective care strategies to reduce hospitalizations and emergency department visits for this vulnerable population. Finally, a concerted effort to identify optimal communication and care planning strategies for this population is needed, particularly surrounding end-of-life decision-making and decision-making surrounding treatment preferences and place of care (Davies et al., 2019). This is particularly true for racial and ethnic communities with belief systems that differ from White western populations, upon which the preponderance of current trials and evidence are based.

More broadly, there is an urgent need to understand and address racial and ethnic disparities in AD/ADRD, serious illness, and multimorbidity. As noted above, there is a higher prevalence of dementia among Black and Latine populations (Quiñones et al., 2020). Research has also indicated disproportionately high AD/ADRD prevalence among the Chamorros, the indigenous people of Guam (Lim et al., 2020). Less is known about disparities among other racial and ethnic groups due to lack of data and underrepresentation in research (Lim et al., 2020; Lin et al., 2022). Racial and ethnic minoritized individuals are less likely to participate in research and clinical trials and recent findings have shown that disparities in dementia incidence can be linked to SDOH, including residential segregation, educational attainment, and occupational complexity, which often stem from structural and systemic racism (Gilmore-Bykovskyi et al., 2019; Pohl et al., 2021). As discussed more extensively in Chapter 4, disparities remain pervasive due to systemic racism, lack of access to care, and discrimination (A. Gilmore-Bykovskyi et al., 2022). To address racial and ethnic disparities for persons living with dementia and multimorbidity, particularly among the seriously ill, future work should prioritize high-quality intervention studies using equity-focused research principles to reduce disparities. Recruitment and retention of diverse participants in dementia research is a priority for improving disparities and developing equitable dementia-focused care.

PALLIATIVE CARE

Palliative care is a specialized interdisciplinary approach to caring for persons living with serious illnesses that focuses on providing a skilled assessment of pain and other symptoms, often in conjunction with delivering comprehensive medical care, providing support and counseling to care partners, and facilitating care coordination while aiming to lessen the stressors of serious illness on patients and their care partners and families (Kelley & Morrison, 2015). Palliative care has been shown to improve symptom burden and quality of life for seriously ill adults across the illness trajectory and often provides the necessary support to meet complex care needs associated with AD/ADRD and multimorbidity (Kavalieratos et al., 2016; Kelley & Morrison, 2015). Documented beneficial outcomes of palliative care include decreased symptom burden, greater care partner support, reduced health care utilization, and completion of advance directives that legally define a patient's wishes regarding life-extending care (Kavalieratos et al., 2016; Quinn et al., 2020). For persons living with dementia, integration of palliative care has been associated with greater likelihood of referral and enrollment in hospice when aligned with goals of care (Lackraj et al., 2021).

Palliative care can be useful for mitigating medical complexity associated with multimorbidity and AD/ADRD (Murali et al., 2020). For example, AD/ADRD and multimorbidity can result in complex symptom burden profiles that require specialized and tailored approaches, which palliative care and serious illness care can provide (Brody et al., 2016). Through tailored pain and symptom management, care coordination, medication management, serious illness communication and planning for end-of-life decision-making regarding care and transitions to hospice, individuals with multimorbidity and AD/ADRD are more likely to receive higher quality of care and experience greater satisfaction with care (Kelley & Morrison, 2015). Palliative care for AD/ADRD also supports the caregiver by facilitating social support services and coordinating the services needed to manage serious illness among patients with multimorbidity.

As with multimorbidity and serious illness, understanding and addressing racial and ethnic disparities in access to palliative care require urgent attention. For example, racially and ethnically minoritized populations are less likely to have adequate pain assessment and treatment, receive goal-concordant care, or complete advance directives (Rhodes et al., 2022). Minoritized individuals are also less likely to receive effective culturally sensitive serious illness communication, an essential component of palliative care (Rhodes et al., 2022). Interventions in palliative care have historically lacked diverse samples, resulting in limited data and a dearth of evidence regarding the serious illness experiences, care needs, preferences, values, and beliefs of racially and ethnically diverse individuals (Jones et al., 2021).

TECHNOLOGY

Rapid advances in technology over the past several decades have encouraged innovation among researchers seeking to improve the health and well-being of patients in a variety of fields, including dementia. Technology-related interventions for people living with AD/ADRD and their care partners have focused principally on improving remote symptom assessment, treatment management, and prevention of falls and serious illness via in-home monitoring, mHealth technology, and electronic health record (EHR)-based interventions (Corbett et al., 2021; O'Brien et al., 2020).

In-Home Monitoring

In-home monitoring typically includes sensors and/or cameras that can be set up around the home to monitor patients for falls and symptoms of illness, creating communication pathways between patients and caregivers when they are off-site. These systems have been taken up rapidly in practice, with even commercially-available, off-the-shelf systems (e.g., Amazon Alexa, Google Home) being adapted for patient monitoring and delivery of services in the home. However, functionality in both commercially-available and research systems does not always live up to the hopes or goals of stakeholders. For instance, systems that require manual input (versus voice) can be challenging for older adults with manual dexterity challenges such as tremors found in Parkinson's Disease and Lewy Body Dementia (Hunter et al., 2020). Additionally, information obtained from remote monitoring systems is not prioritized in primary care providers' overflowing EHR inboxes, leading to a false sense of security and risk of missed early intervention (Shah et al., 2019). In addition, challenges related to patient acceptability, privacy, usability, and cost persist (Holthe et al., 2018). With the rapid advances in technology and breaking down of hesitancy around technology due to privacy concerns, some of these viewpoints and challenges are rapidly receding from public view, even if they still exist and need further addressing for both ethical, safety, and equity considerations (Ozeran et al., 2021).

In addition to general in-home monitoring systems, more scientifically-advanced remote physiologic monitoring (RPM) and remote therapeutic monitoring (RTM) systems allow for technology to be used in the home for health care systems and providers to monitor patients and receive reimbursement from insurers. RPM and RTM systems can be used to obtain physiologic measurements remotely, such as blood pressure or blood sugar readings; they can also be used to support symptom control and medication adherence (Kruklitis et al., 2022). While these systems are still in relative infancy, challenges to their wider adoption include ensuring the technologies are easily usable by diverse patient populations, including older adults and those with dementia; provide multi-language support for patients with limited English proficiency; and can be integrated effectively into EHRs, so that data becomes part of the patient record and portal and can be reviewed and acted upon by health care providers. Most RPM and RTM systems have not yet met these requirements. However, incentivized by high levels of reimbursement, these systems are gaining traction among health care providers. To realize their potential among the diverse population of people living with dementia, developers will need to tailor tools to meet the needs of racially, culturally, and linguistically diverse people living with AD/ADRD and their care partners.

mHealth Technology

The constellation of technological solutions referred to as mHealth technology includes a wide array of sophisticated smart phone apps alongside simpler technologies such as SMS text messaging. In recent years, access to smart phones has increased across individuals of all racial, ethnic, and socioeconomic backgrounds, in part due to the availability of subsidies for low-income Americans (Yousaf et al., 2020). In parallel, the use of mHealth technology has also grown substantially; the number of apps has grown from 66,000 in 2013 to over 350,000 in 2021 (IQVIA, 2021). While use among persons living with dementia and their care partners within this group is small, it is growing and best practices have been developed for usability (Engelsma et al., 2021).

One of the significant benefits of mHealth technology is that it can be created dynamically to personalize choices and messages for the intended recipient. Health-related technological systems may focus on a set of patient attributes to encourage adoption of behavior change with reminders and push notifications in much the same way that a commercial retailer may target advertising and notifications to a consumer seeking a specific pair of shoes or clothing (Montag et al., 2020). By employing behavioral economics principles, these systems can better tailor strategies to patient attributes and preferences, motivating individuals to perform certain actions by using specific phrasing, language, and defaults

(Thorgeirsson & Kawachi, 2013). One commonly employed aspect of behavioral economics within mHealth is gamification, which refers to the strategic use of game design elements to improve user engagement and motivate individuals. For example, for individuals using an mHealth app to increase their physical activity, the program may use a leaderboard to display the ranking of individuals to encourage friendly competition or a badge system to recognize achievement. Gamification could help care partners to engage in mHealth systems to improve uptake of data collection, intervention implementation, or medication adherence, among other possibilities.

EHRs

EHRs are in common use throughout US health care institutions and offer important tools for treatment management, tracking of patient outcomes, patient–provider communication, and coordination of care among different care partners and organizations involved in the social and medical support of patients with chronic conditions, including AD/ADRD. As discussed in Chapter 6, EHRs can also be instrumental in expanding clinical research participation by understudied groups, including racial and ethnic minoritized populations. Particularly for patients living with dementia who have comorbidities, EHRs allow care partners to have greater connection with the health system, facilitating scheduling, tracking health outcomes such as lab values, and communicating with the clinical team. These systems also can serve clinicians by providing best practice alerts or other clinical decision support to nudge toward best practice or implementing predictive analytic algorithms to identify those at risk of certain conditions or poor outcomes.

However, realizing the promise of EHRs for people living with AD/ADRD is challenging. At the most fundamental level, system interoperability must be addressed. Entering data into EHRs may be relatively easy but using and sharing data among clinicians to foster engagement and attention across a multidisciplinary care team is considerably more difficult – whether within a single institution or across several organizations. Many technologies lack the ability to "flag" concerning symptoms or problems for clinicians due to the limitations of existing interoperability standards. While customized flags can be created in individual systems, they require programming time and implementation on an organizational basis. Moreover, although EHRs are in use by most health care practices, different companies' products cannot necessarily "talk" to each other; in parallel, the mHealth apps discussed in the section above may lack a common language for communicating with EHRs, rendering their promise unfulfilled. There is much work to do to find the best pathways for flagging concerns raised by mHealth within EHRs while also limiting overwhelming inputs and messages for time-constrained primary care providers and teams who perform substantial amounts of uncompensated care (Sinsky et al., 2022).

With respect to persons living with dementia, critical questions persist about how to include care partners and caregivers within the EHR. While parents are often provided "proxy access" to their children's records, caregivers of adults with dementia typically do not have the same access. Furthermore, EHRs do not accommodate loss of capacity among patients with dementia; that is, these systems do not encompass options for management of personal health information (PHI) as the health of these patients deteriorates. There is a need for systemic efforts to develop and integrate protocols for involving care partners early in the process, when patients with dementia are able to understand the likely trajectory of their illness and give consent for their care partners to view and act upon their PHI. At present, many health centers do not know how to provide proxy access to care partners in order to allow them to view the patients' EHR. Thus, care partners must either seek "work-arounds," such as using the patient's login to the portal in order to view test results and interact with providers online; or they have no access at all to critical health data. These fundamental system-based challenges can be further exacerbated by systematic bias, racism, limited technology access and literacy, limited English proficiency, and classism – all of which contribute to mistrust among providers, patients, and care partners and may negatively impact the involvement of the care partner in the patient's care, leading to poorer outcomes.

Further, while emergency contacts are included prominently within the patient's health record, care partners and other caregivers usually are not. This missing data impacts research recruitment and clinical trial participation. Within this context, when dementia researchers seek appropriate research participants from within a health care institution's EHR, difficulties in contacting patients and locating the care partner to participate in dyadic research may prove insurmountably challenging. Even when the care partner or caregiver is listed in the EHR, unless that person is also a patient within the same health system, regulatory and legal obstacles may prevent providers from reaching out to these people directly. In practice, when providers need to discuss treatment with the care partners, this distinction may be ignored; however, in the context of research, the lack of a legal framework allowing for outreach to care partners can prevent researchers from including a diverse group of patients and care partners in their study pool, if not derail study recruitment and implementation altogether.

Addressing Challenges in Future Research

In addition to the challenges described above, numerous considerations must be woven into the design of research seeking to develop technological support for persons living with dementia and their care partners (Table 9.1).

TABLE 9.1 Challenges to Implementation of Health Care Technology Solutions for Persons Living with Dementia

- Differential access to broadband, wireless technology, computers, and smart phones (Pew Research Center, 2021).
- Persons living with dementia may experience visual or hearing impairment, resulting in unfamiliarity with technology and difficulties in use (Wildenbos et al., 2018).
- Privacy and confidentiality concerns may limit use (Kao & Liebovitz, 2017).
- Some forms of technology (e.g., smart phone apps and EHRs) may lack interoperability and/or the capability for meaningful and useful data extraction and sharing among clinicians (Kao & Liebovitz, 2017).
- Few end users from minoritized and underserved groups or with limited English proficiency have participated in technological research, contributing to increased racial and ethnic disparities in technology use (Anderson-Lewis et al., 2018).

Future work needs to address tailoring toward diverse populations with varying levels of technical literacy. Additional work needs to address how the care partner is included within health systems and electronic health records, and in how to create sustainable systems for flagging or monitoring of persons living with dementia or care partner generated data so that the onus does not lie solely on them to intervene with the clinical team, which can create significant health disparities based on level of comfort with advocating, cultural differences, and health literacy levels.

SUMMARY

While there are many emerging areas in AD/ADRD care, the four represented herein – i.e., dyadic and caregiving, multimorbidity and serious illness, palliative care, and technology – represent significant areas of study that have been growing but still have substantial need for development. Additionally, each of these four areas intersectionally interact with health equity concerns, particularly around access and issues of systematic racism and bias. Therefore, there is a need within the AD/ADRD research community to perform research that purposefully recruits diverse participants for clinical and community trials as well as implements research exclusively within minoritized groups that is not comparative but focuses on individual racial and ethnic communities to understand and respond to their unique attributes and specific needs.

DISCUSSION QUESTIONS

1. What are some benefits and challenges to consider when conducting dyadic research with persons living with dementia and their care partners?

2. What are some examples of complex care needs among persons living with dementia and multimorbidity?

3. What are some of the barriers to implementing technology-informed interventions in diverse communities and how do we consider equity in the development and implementation of technology of interventions?

REFERENCES

Aldridge, M. D., Hunt, L., Husain, M., Li, L., & Kelley, A. (2022). Impact of Comorbid Dementia on patterns of hospice use. *Journal of Palliative Medicine*, *25*(3), 396–404. https://doi.org/10.1089/jpm.2021.0055

Alzheimer's Association. (2022). 2022 Alzheimer's disease facts and figures. *Alzheimer's & Dementia*, *18*(4), 700–789. https://doi.org/https://doi.org/10.1002/alz.12638

Amjad, H., Snyder, S. H., Wolff, J. L., Oh, E., & Samus, Q. M. (2019). Before hospice: Symptom Burden, Dementia, and social participation in the last year of life. *Journal of Palliative Medicine*, *22*(9), 1106–1114. https://doi.org/10.1089/jpm.2018.0479

Anderson-Lewis, C., Darville, G., Mercado, R. E., Howell, S., & Di Maggio, S. (2018). mHealth technology use and implications in historically underserved and minority populations in the United States: Systematic literature review. *JMIR Mhealth Uhealth*, *6*(6), e128. https://doi.org/10.2196/mhealth.8383

Bonds Johnson, K., Brewster, G. S., Cicero, E., Hepburn, K., Clevenger, C. K., Daniel, G., Pak, V., Paul, S., & Epps, F. (2021). Promoting caregiver mastery in black American Dementia caregivers. *Gerontologist*, *62*(5). https://doi.org/10.1093/geront/gnab147

Bonds Johnson, K., Epps, F. R., Song, M., Lyons, K. S., & Driessnack, M. (2021). Using poetry as data to explore daily and formal care decision making within African American dementia dyads. *Geriatric Nursing, 42*(4), 919–925. https://doi.org/10.1016/j.gerinurse.2021.05.001

Bonds, K., Whitlatch, C. J., Song, M., & Lyons, K. S. (2020). Factors influencing quality of life in African-American dementia dyads. *Aging & Mental Health, 25*(4), 1–8. https://doi.org/10.1080/13607863.2020.1711865

Brody, A. A., Guan, C., Cortes, T., & Galvin, J. E. (2016). Development and testing of the Dementia symptom management at home (DSM-H) program: An interprofessional home health care intervention to improve the quality of life for persons with dementia and their caregivers. *Geriatric Nursing (New York, N.Y.), 37*(3), 200–206. https://doi.org/10.1016/j.gerinurse.2016.01.002

Burgdorf, J. G., Arbaje, A. I., Stuart, E. A., & Wolff, J. L. (2021). Unmet family caregiver training needs associated with acute care utilization during home health care. *Journal of the American Geriatrics Society, 69*(7), 1887–1895. https://doi.org/10.1111/jgs.17138

Cook, W. L., & Kenny, D. A. (2005). The Actor–Partner Interdependence Model: A model of bidirectional effects in developmental studies. *International Journal of Behavioral Development, 29*(2), 101–109. https://doi.org/10.1080/01650250444000405

Corbett, C. F., Combs, E. M., Chandarana, P. S., Stringfellow, I., Worthy, K., Nguyen, T., Wright, P. J., & O'Kane, J. M. (2021). Medication adherence reminder system for virtual home assistants: Mixed methods evaluation study. *JMIR Formative Research, 5*(7), e27327. https://doi.org/10.2196/27327

Davies, N., Schiowitz, B., Rait, G., Vickerstaff, V., & Sampson, E. L. (2019). Decision aids to support decision-making in dementia care: A systematic review. *International Psychogeriatrics, 31*(10), 1403–1419. https://doi.org/10.1017/S1041610219000826

Engelsma, T., Jaspers, M. W. M., & Peute, L. W. (2021). Considerate mHealth design for older adults with Alzheimer's disease and related dementias (ADRD): A scoping review on usability barriers and design suggestions. *International Journal of Medical Informatics, 152,* 104494. https://doi.org/10.1016/j.ijmedinf.2021.104494

Gilmore-Bykovskyi, A., Croff, R., Glover, C. M., Jackson, J. D., Resendez, J., Perez, A., Zuelsdorff, M., Green-Harris, G., & Manly, J. J. (2022). Traversing the aging research and health equity divide: Toward intersectional frameworks of research justice and participation. *The Gerontologist, 62*(5), 711–720. https://doi.org/10.1093/geront/gnab107

Gilmore-Bykovskyi, A. L., Jin, Y., Gleason, C., Flowers-Benton, S., Block, L. M., Dilworth-Anderson, P., Barnes, L. L., Shah, M. N., & Zuelsdorff, M. (2019). Recruitment and retention of underrepresented populations in Alzheimer's disease research: A systematic review. *Alzheimer's & Dementia (New York, N. Y.), 5*(1), 751–770. https://doi.org/10.1016/j.trci.2019.09.018

Gilmore-Bykovskyi, A. L., Roberts, T. J., King, B. J., Kennelty, K. A., & Kind, A. J. H. (2017). Transitions from hospitals to skilled nursing facilities for persons with dementia: A challenging convergence of patient and system-level needs. *The Gerontologist, 57*(5), 867–879. https://doi.org/10.1093/geront/gnw085

Grembowski, D., Schaefer, J., Johnson, K., Fischer, H., Moore, S., Tai-Seale, M., Ricciardi, R., Fraser, J., Miller, D., & LeRoy, L. (2014). A conceptual model of the role of complexity in the care of patients with multiple chronic conditions. *Medical Care, 52*(Suppl 3), S7–S14. Suppl 2, *ADVANCING THE FIELD: Results from the AHRQ Multiple Chronic Conditions Research Network* (3). https://doi.org/10.1097/MLR.0000000000000045

Harrison, K. L., Ritchie, C. S., Hunt, L. J., Patel, K., Boscardin, W. J., Yaffe, K., & Smith, A. K. (2022). Life expectancy for community-dwelling persons with dementia and severe disability. *Journal of the American Geriatrics Society, 70*(6), 1807–1815. https://doi.org/10.1111/jgs.17767

Holthe, T., Halvorsrud, L., Karterud, D., Hoel, K. A., & Lund, A. (2018). Usability and acceptability of technology for community-dwelling older adults with mild cognitive impairment and dementia: A systematic literature review. *Clinical Interventions in Aging, 13,* 863–886. https://doi.org/10.2147/CIA.S154717

Hu, M., Ma, C., Sadarangani, T., & Wu, B. (2021). Social-behavioral interventions for Asian and Hispanic American dementia caregivers: An integrative review. *Aging and Health Research, 1*(3). https://doi.org/10.1016/j.ahr.2021.100027

Hunter, I., Elers, P., Lockhart, C., Guesgen, H., Singh, A., & Whiddett, D. (2020). Issues associated with the management and governance of sensor data and information to assist aging in place: Focus group study with health care professionals. *JMIR mHealth and uHealth, 8*(12), e24157. https://doi.org/10.2196/24157

IQVIA. (2021). Digital health trends 2021. Available at: https://www.iqvia.com/insights/the-iqvia-institute/reports/digital-health-trends-2021#. Accessed December 19, 2022

Jones, T., Luth, E. A., Lin, S., & Brody, A. A. (2021). Advance care planning, palliative care, and end-of-life care interventions for racial and ethnic underrepresented groups: A systematic review. *Journal of Pain and Symptom Management, 62*(3), e248–e260. https://doi.org/10.1016/j.jpainsymman.2021.04.025

Kao, C. K., & Liebovitz, D. M. (2017). Consumer mobile health apps: Current state, barriers, and future directions. *PM & R: The Journal of Injury, Function, and Rehabilitation, 9*(5S), S106–S115. https://doi.org/10.1016/j.pmrj.2017.02.018

Kavalieratos, D., Corbelli, J., Zhang, D., Dionne-Odom, J. N., Ernecoff, N. C., Hanmer, J., Hoydich, Z. P., Ikejiani, D. Z., Klein-Fedyshin, M., Zimmermann, C., Morton, S. C., Arnold, R. M., Heller, L., & Schenker, Y. (2016). Association between palliative care and patient and caregiver outcomes: A systematic review and meta-analysis. *JAMA, 316*(20), 2104–2114. https://doi.org/10.1001/jama.2016.16840

Kelley, A. S. (2014). Defining "serious illness". *Journal of Palliative Medicine, 17*(9), 985. https://doi.org/10.1089/jpm.2014.0164

Kelley, A. S., & Morrison, R. S. (2015). Palliative care for the seriously Ill. *The New England Journal of Medicine, 373*(8), 747–755. https://doi.org/10.1056/NEJMra1404684

Kruklitis, R., Miller, M., Valeriano, L., Shine, S., Opstbaum, N., & Chestnut, V. (2022). Applications of remote patient monitoring. *Primary Care; Clinics in Office Practice, 49*(4), 543–555. https://doi.org/10.1016/j.pop.2022.05.005

Lackraj, D., Kavalieratos, D., Murali, K. P., Lu, Y., & Hua, M. (2021). Implementation of specialist palliative care and outcomes for hospitalized patients with dementia. *Journal of the American Geriatrics Society, 69*(5), 1199–1207. https://doi.org/10.1111/jgs.17032

Lim, S., Mohaimin, S., Min, D., Roberts, T., Sohn, Y. J., Wong, J., Sivanesathurai, R., Kwon, S. C., & Trinh-Shevrin, C. (2020). Alzheimer's disease and its related dementias among Asian Americans, Native Hawaiians, and Pacific Islanders: A scoping review. *Journal of Alzheimer's Disease: JAD, 77*(2), 523–537. https://doi.org/10.3233/JAD-200509

Lin, P., Zhu, Y., Olchanski, N., Cohen, J. T., Neumann, P. J., Faul, J. D., Fillit, H. M., & Freund, K. M. (2022). Racial and ethnic differences in hospice use and hospitalizations at End-of-Life among medicare beneficiaries with dementia. *JAMA Network Open, 5*(6), e2216260. https://doi.org/10.1001/jamanetworkopen.2022.16260

Lyons, K. S., & Lee, C. S. (2020). A multilevel modeling approach to examine incongruent illness appraisals in family care dyads over time. *Journal of Family Nursing, 26*(3). https://doi.org/10.1177/1074840720944439

Lyons, K. S., Zarit, S. H., Sayer, A. G., & Whitlatch, C. J. (2002). Caregiving as a dyadic process: Perspectives from caregiver and receiver [Article]. *Journals of Gerontology - Series B Psychological Sciences and Social Sciences, 57*(3), P195–P204. https://doi.org/10.1093/geronb/57.3.P195

Makoul, G., & Clayman, M. L. (2006). An integrative model of shared decision making in medical encounters. *Patient Education and Counseling, 60*(3), 301–312. https://doi.org/10.1016/j.pec.2005.06.010

Maust, D. T., Kales, H. C., McCammon, R. J., Blow, F. C., Leggett, A., & Langa, K. M. (2017). Distress associated with dementia-related psychosis and agitation in relation to healthcare utilization and costs. *The American Journal of Geriatric Psychiatry: Official Journal of the American Association for Geriatric Psychiatry, 25*(10), 1074–1082. https://doi.org/10.1016/j.jagp.2017.02.025

Maust, D. T., Kim, H. M., Chiang, C., Langa, K. M., & Kales, H. C. (2019). Predicting risk of potentially preventable hospitalization in older adults with dementia. *Journal of the American Geriatrics Society, 67*(10), 2077–2084. https://doi.org/10.1111/jgs.16030

Mitchell, S. L. (2015). Advanced dementia. *The New England Journal of Medicine, 373*(13), 1276–1277. https://doi.org/10.1056/NEJMc1509349

Mitchell, S. L., Teno, J. M., Kiely, D. K., Shaffer, M. L., Jones, R. N., Prigerson, H. G., Volicer, L., Givens, J. L., & Hamel, M. B. (2009). The clinical course of advanced dementia. *The New England Journal of Medicine, 361*(16), 1529–1538. https://doi.org/10.1056/NEJMoa0902234

Montag, C., Sindermann, C., & Baumeister, H. (2020). Digital phenotyping in psychological and medical sciences: A reflection about necessary prerequisites to reduce harm and increase benefits. *Current Opinion in Psychology, 36*, 19–24. https://doi.org/10.1016/j.copsyc.2020.03.013

Murali, K. P., Kang, J. A., Bronstein, D., McDonald, M. V., King, L., Chastain, A. M., & Shang, J. (2022). Measuring palliative care-related knowledge, attitudes, and confidence in home health care clinicians, patients, and caregivers: A systematic review. *Journal of Palliative Medicine.* https://doi.org/10.1089/jpm.2021.0580

Murali, K. P., Merriman, J. D., Yu, G., Vorderstrasse, A., Kelley, A., & Brody, A. A. (2020). An adapted conceptual model integrating palliative care in serious illness and multiple chronic conditions. *The American Journal of Hospice & Palliative Care, 37*(12), 1086–1095. https://doi.org/10.1177/1049909120928353

Murali, K. P., Yu, G., Merriman, J. D., Vorderstrasse, A., Kelley, A. S., & Brody, A. A. (2021). Multiple chronic conditions among seriously ill adults receiving palliative care. *Western Journal of Nursing Research*, 1939459211041174. https://doi.org/10.1177/01939459211041174

National Academy of Sciences. (2021). Reducing the impact of dementia in America: A decadal survey of the behavioral and social sciences. National Academies Press (US).

O'Brien, K., Liggett, A., Ramirez-Zohfeld, V., Sunkara, P., & Lindquist, L. A. (2020). Voice-controlled intelligent personal assistants to support aging in place. *Journal of the American Geriatrics Society*, 68(1), 176–179. https://doi.org/10.1111/jgs.16217

Ozeran, L., Solomonides, A., & Schreiber, R. (2021). Privacy versus convenience: A historical perspective, analysis of risks, and an informatics call to action. *Applied Clinical Informatics*, 12(2), 274–284. https://doi.org/10.1055/s-0041-1727197

Parker, L. J., Gaugler, J. E., & Gitlin, L. N. (2022). Use of critical race theory to inform the recruitment of Black/African American Alzheimer's disease caregivers into community-based research. *The Gerontologist*, 62(5), 742–750. https://doi.org/10.1093/geront/gnac001

Pew Research Center. (2021). Internet/Broadband Fact Sheet. https://www.pewresearch.org/internet/fact-sheet/internet-broadband

Ploeg, J., Northwood, M., Duggleby, W., McAiney, C. A., Chambers, T., Peacock, S., Fisher, K., Ghosh, S., Markle-Reid, M., Swindle, J., Williams, A., & Triscott, J. A. (2020). Caregivers of older adults with dementia and multiple chronic conditions: Exploring their experiences with significant changes. *Dementia (London, England)*, 19(8), 2601–2620. https://doi.org/10.1177/1471301219834423

Pohl, D. J., Seblova, D., Avila, J. F., Dorsman, K. A., Kulick, E. R., Casey, J. A., & Manly, J. (2021). Relationship between residential segregation, later-life cognition, and incident dementia across race/ethnicity. *International Journal of Environmental Research and Public Health*, 18(21). https://doi.org/10.3390/ijerph182111233

Quinn, K. L., Shurrab, M., Gitau, K., Kavalieratos, D., Isenberg, S. R., Stall, N. M., Stukel, T. A., Goldman, R., Horn, D., Cram, P., Detsky, A. S., & Bell, C. M. (2020). Association of receipt of palliative care interventions with health care use, quality of life, and symptom burden among adults with chronic noncancer illness: A systematic review and meta-analysis. *Jama*, 324(14), 1439–1450. https://doi.org/10.1001/jama.2020.14205

Quiñones, A. R., Kaye, J., Allore, H. G., Botoseneanu, A., & Thielke, S. M. (2020). An agenda for addressing multimorbidity and racial and ethnic disparities in Alzheimer's Disease and related dementia. *American Journal of Alzheimer's Disease and Other Dementias*, 35 1533317520960874. https://doi.org/10.1177/1533317520960874

Rhodes, R. L., Barrett, N. J., Ejem, D. B., Sloan, D. H., Bullock, K., Bethea, K., Durant, R. W., Anderson, G. T., Hasan, M., Travitz, G., Thompson, A., & Johnson, K. S. (2022). A review of race and ethnicity in hospice and palliative medicine research: Representation matters. *Journal of Pain and Symptom Management*, 64(5), e289–e299. https://doi.org/10.1016/j.jpainsymman.2022.07.009

Sadarangani, T., Perissinotto, C., Boafo, J., Zhong, J., & Yu, G. (2022). Multimorbidity patterns in adult day health center clients with dementia: A latent class analysis. *BMC Geriatrics*, 22(1), 514. https://doi.org/10.1186/s12877-022-03206-0

Sebern, M. D., & Whitlatch, C. J. (2007). Dyadic relationship scale: A measure of the impact of the provision and receipt of family care [Article]. *Gerontologist*, 47(6), 741–751. https://doi.org/10.1093/geront/47.6.741

Shay, L. A., & Lafata, J. E. (2015). Where is the evidence? A systematic review of shared decision making and patient outcomes. *Medical Decision Making*, 35(1), 114–131. https://doi.org/10.1177/0272989x14551638

Shah, T., Patel-Teague, S., Kroupa, L., Meyer, A. N. D., & Singh, H. (2019). Impact of a national QI programme on reducing electronic health record notifications to clinicians. *BMJ Quality and Safety*, 28(1), 10–14. https://doi.org/10.1136/bmjqs-2017-007447

Shin, J. Y., & Habermann, B. (2022). Caregivers of adults living with Alzheimer's Disease or dementia in 2020: A secondary analysis. *Journal of Gerontological Nursing*, 48(9), 15–25. https://doi.org/10.3928/00989134-20220805-02

Sinsky, C. A., Shanafelt, T. D., & Ripp, J. A. (2022). The electronic health record inbox: Recommendations for relief. *Journal of General Internal Medicine*, 37(15), 4002–4003. https://doi.org/10.1007/s11606-022-07766-0

Sisco, S., Gross, A. L., Shih, R. A., Sachs, B. C., Glymour, M. M., Bangen, K. J., Benitez, A., Skinner, J., Schneider, B. C., & Manly, J. J. (2015). The role of early-life educational quality and literacy in explaining racial disparities in cognition in late life. *Journals of Gerontology B Psychological Sciences and Social Science*, 70(4), 557–567. https://doi.org/10.1093/geronb/gbt133

Snowden, M. B., Steinman, L. E., Bryant, L. L., Cherrier, M. M., Greenlund, K. J., Leith, K. H., Levy, C., Logsdon, R. G., Copeland, C., Vogel, M., Anderson, L. A., Atkins, D. C., Bell, J. F., & Fitzpatrick, A. L. (2017). Dementia and co-occurring chronic conditions: A systematic literature review to identify what is known and where are the gaps in the evidence? *International Journal of Geriatric Psychiatry*, *32*(4), 357–371. https://doi.org/10.1002/gps.4652

Szabo, S. M., Whitlatch, C. J., Orsulic-Jeras, S., & Johnson, J. D. (2016). Recruitment challenges and strategies: Lessons learned from an early-stage dyadic intervention (innovative practice). *Dementia (London)*. https://doi.org/10.1177/1471301216659608

Ta Park, V., Grill, J. D., Zhu, J., Nguyen, K., Nam, B., Tsoh, J., Kanaya, A., Vuong, Q., Bang, J., Nguyen, N. C. Y., Cho, I. H., Gallagher-Thompson, D., Hinton, L., & Meyer, O. L. (2021). Asian Americans and Pacific Islanders' perspectives on participating in the CARE recruitment research registry for Alzheimer's disease and related dementias, aging, and caregiving research. *Alzheimer's & Dementia (New York, N. Y.)*, *7*(1), e12195. https://doi.org/10.1002/trc2.12195

Thorgeirsson, T., & Kawachi, I. (2013). Behavioral economics: Merging psychology and economics for lifestyle interventions. *American Journal of Preventive Medicine*, *44*(2), 185–189. https://doi.org/10.1016/j.amepre.2012.10.008

Whitlatch, C. J., Judge, K., Zarit, S. H., & Femia, E. (2006). Dyadic intervention for family caregivers and care receivers in early-stage dementia. *Gerontologist*, *46*(5), 688–694. https://doi.org/10.1093/geront/46.5.688

Wildenbos, G. A., Peute, L., & Jaspers, M. (2018). Aging barriers influencing mobile health usability for older adults: A literature based framework (MOLD-US). *International Journal of Medical Informatics*, *114*, 66–75. https://doi.org/10.1016/j.ijmedinf.2018.03.012

Yousaf, K., Mehmood, Z., Awan, I. A., Saba, T., Alharbey, R., Qadah, T., & Alrige, M. A. (2020). A comprehensive study of mobile-health based assistive technology for the healthcare of dementia and Alzheimer's disease (AD). *Health Care Management Science*, *23*(2), 287–309. https://doi.org/10.1007/s10729-019-09486-0

INDEX

Please note that page references to tables are followed by the letter "t".

Population Science Methods and Approaches to Aging and Alzheimer's Disease and Related Dementias Research, First Edition. Edited by Chau Trinh-Shevrin.
© 2024 John Wiley & Sons, Inc. Published 2024 by John Wiley & Sons, Inc.

health-promoting behaviors, 22
health services research (HSR), 81
heavy metals, 21
HIV/AIDS, 46, 51–53
homophobic policies, 51
human capital, 95
hybrid designs, 81
hypertension, 5, 37

I

immigrants,
  cognitive assessment and diagnosis in, 36, 52
  and cognitive decline, 30
  and economic stability, 18
  and family support, 49
  and health inequities, 3–4
  and mental health, 7
implementation outcomes, 80, 84–85
Implementation Outcomes
      Framework (IOF), 85
implementation research, 79, 86–87
implementation science (IS), 77–86
  key terms and definitions, 79–81
  theories and frameworks, 82–83
implementation strategies, 79–80, 83–84
incarceration, 35–36
in-home monitoring, 131–132
injustice, 3
insomnia, 108–109, 116
Institute of Medicine (IOM), 81
institutional review board (IRB), 68
intersectionality, 46–47, 51–53
intervention mapping, 84
IOF see Implementation Outcomes Framework
IRB see institutional review board
IS see implementation science

J

Japanese Americans, 22
Jim Crow laws, 32
job strain, 34–35

K

Korean Americans, 5

L

Langford, Aisha T., 64

language, 67
  see also limited English proficiency (LEP)
Latine people,
  access to health care, 19–20, 35
  COVID-19, 8, 9
  demographic trends, 2
  educational achievement, 33
  food insecurity, 8, 21
  health status, 3, 4
  income and economic stability, 18
  LGBTQ+, 52
  mental health, 7
  occupational hazards, 34
  perceptions of aging, 5
  prevalence of AD/ADRD, 4, 6, 127
  research participation, 61
  residential segregation, 32
  sleep health, 115–116
LEP see limited English proficiency
LGBTQ+ people, 45–54
  caregiver stress, 49–51, 53
  and discrimination, 47–49, 53
  health disparities, 46, 52
  mental health, 7
  prevalence of dementia, 46
  racial and ethnic minority, 52–53
  and social isolation, 49–51
life expectancy, 3, 52, 108
limited English proficiency (LEP), 3, 6, 8, 21
literacy, 33, 34, 65
loneliness, 7
  see also social isolation

M

malnutrition, 8
Medicare, 48
medication, 35
memory, 33
men,
  Black, 52
  gay and bisexual, 47, 52
mental health, 7, 53, 112–113
mental illness, 52, 53
metabolic waste hypothesis, 113
Mexican Americans, 32
mHealth technology, 132–133
military, 50
Mini-Mental State Examination, 36
mobility, 61, 111